How to Sleep Like a Caveman

How to Sleep Like a Caveman

Ancient Wisdom for a Better Night's Rest

Merijn van de Laar

WILLIAM
COLLINS

William Collins
An imprint of HarperCollins*Publishers*
1 London Bridge Street
London SE1 9GF

WilliamCollinsBooks.com

HarperCollins*Publishers*
Macken House
39/40 Mayor Street Upper
Dublin 1
D01 C9W8, Ireland

First published in Great Britain in 2025 by William Collins

1

ISBN 978-0-00-871761-2 (hardback)
ISBN 978-0-00-871762-9 (trade paperback)

Typeset in Adobe Garamond Pro by Jouve (UK), Milton Keynes

Printed and bound in Great Britain by CPI Group (UK) Ltd, Croydon

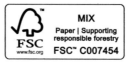

In loving memory of Alda and Noa

Contents

Contents

Contents

Introduction

Sleep is a magical phenomenon. When you are a good sleeper, you close your eyes and, before you know it, you go on a journey into a wonderful world beyond full consciousness. If you sleep poorly, the night can feel like a punishment. Every night becomes a struggle with yourself, often leading to negative thoughts and feelings of helplessness. And once the sun comes up, you dread the day which seems endless. Concentration and memory problems, mood swings and a lack of energy can result from the nightly struggles.

While working as a sleep therapist, I researched the causes of insomnia. In my consultation room I was sometimes amazed at how great the individual differences in the perception of sleep were. I met people who could barely put one foot in front of the other after 7 hours of sleep, but also clients who got through the day just fine on 5 hours. Some in the latter group did not even think of themselves as having a sleep problem but had partners who thought otherwise. The subjective experience of sleep and sleep problems appeared to be an important but somewhat elusive factor in their various daytime and night-time impairments.

Because of these experiences, I embarked on scientific research with the aim of unravelling some of the secrets of sleep. In particular, I wanted to examine what psychological factors play a role in sleep problems. My patients often expressed night-time worries about not sleeping enough and demonstrated accompanying feelings of help-lessness. Could specific personality traits explain these experiences? Are these individuals perhaps more perfectionist or compulsive? Do they worry more in general or display more anxiousness?

Fortunately, insomniacs turned out to be no different in their personalities from people without insomnia. I say fortunately, because I was secretly pleased with that finding. After all, I myself have known long periods of poor sleep, and I like the idea that I'm not too different because of it.

My sleep problems started at a very early age. As a baby, I slept poorly. My mother suffered from tiredness after spending many nights awake because of my cries. In desperation, she decided to visit the family doctor, who referred me to hospital for two days of observations. There I slept like a rock from the very first night. However, once I got home, I was constantly crying again. The doctors and nurses finally advised: 'Just let the little man cry it out, he'll fall asleep by himself.' That turned out to work well and I slept fine for years afterwards. In hindsight, the hospital practised the cry-it-out method, which focuses on letting the baby cry without any intervention and teaches the child to calm itself down and fall asleep alone. Nowadays, this method is controversial according to some, but at the time it worked well for me.

At age 28, things went wrong. I was working as a therapist at a sleep centre, and I was once again plagued by bad nights. It took hours to fall asleep and I woke up every hour, watching the time pass by on my alarm clock. During the night, I had repetitive negative thoughts about my expected malfunction the next day and about how miserable I would feel again at work. I felt deeply embarrassed: during the day I treated people with insomnia, and at night I lay awake myself. I did not follow my own sleep recommendations. I felt like a pulmonologist who advises his patients not to smoke and then secretly lights a cigarette himself. I could not figure out why I was suddenly sleeping so badly, and found it difficult to accept.

A month later, my family doctor referred me to a psychotherapist. At first I was uncomfortable with the sessions: I literally sat with my back to him while he asked questions about my childhood. Nevertheless, after a few sessions I began to sleep better; it also helped that a colleague in the sleep centre encouraged me to apply certain aspects of the sleep therapy I gave to patients to myself. The idea that I could suddenly develop a sleep problem puzzled me. I started looking for the mechanisms of good sleep. I wanted to understand why regular sleep treatments do not work for everyone.

An understanding of the onset of my sleeplessness came only years later when I discovered that basic processes, developed in early human evolution, had been hampering my night's rest. Next to being surprised, the idea that something from ancient times could explain many current sleep theories sparked my curiosity. I already had a strong interest in evolution, dating from my late teens when I studied psychology. Though I'd found many aspects of my course boring, the evolutionary psychology modules had created a strong urge in me to learn more about the topic. I was excited to discover that we have lost knowledge about how our bodies function in natural circumstances, and to find that evolutionary principles can explain the expression of emotions such as fear, anger and sadness.

Many years later, when I worked as a sleep therapist, I discovered that lying awake does not necessarily have to be a bad thing, because ancient humans probably lay awake more than we did. However, the way you lie awake is important, which I will tell you more about later. It likely made sense to be awake longer and more often if there was a nocturnal threat from predators or hostile tribes. In this way, you and your tribe could respond more quickly and get to safety. Moreover, I realised that to understand the nature of sleep, we must go back to prehistoric times, when our bodies were far more adapted to natural conditions through evolution. What did primeval humans do to get a good night's rest? What did our primal sleep look like? Did cave dwellers always take care of their sleep, or did they sometimes engage in sleep-interfering activities such as substance use? Did they experience worries or fears around sleep? What did they eat and how did their diet affect their sleep?

This book will give answers to questions such as why evolution might have led to better sleep in people who fall in love, why sex might help us fall asleep, and how a good night's rest makes us more attractive. What is the relationship between ancient nocturnal predators and modern worries, and what is the effect of mood on sleep, and vice versa? I will discuss the function of dreams, fragmented sleep and other night-time experiences, such as sleepwalking. What role do dreams play in our emotions and how could they have helped *Homo sapiens* survive through millennia? I will discuss the effect of stimulants on sleep. Moreover, what about sleep medication? What exactly does it do to our slumber? This book also focuses on the effect of sleep on mortality, health and chronic disease. How can we keep ourselves healthy?

Many books tell you about things you should do and not do in order to promote sleep. They give you all kinds of tips on how to think, how to behave and even how to feel. Those tips often help, even if you don't understand why. In this book I want to go a step further and help you understand more about restful nights, why you need them and why you are a good or a bad sleeper. By zooming in on how we probably lived hundreds of thousands of years ago, I hope to give insights into what the evolutionary background of sleep is and how you can use this for your own benefit. I also want to debunk several unhelpful myths around our night's rest. An example is the 8-hour myth, which is not in line with evidence from research on the probable lives of our ancestors. While doing this, I want to give comfort to people who currently suffer from sleeplessness, help them to sleep better, and to be more relaxed when they are awake at night.

Note: This book mainly discusses normal sleep and sleep problems which are responsive to (cognitive) behavioural interventions, namely: insomnia, delayed sleep phase syndrome, and parasomnia. Sleep disorders such as sleep apnoea and narcolepsy are not the main scope of this work; if you suspect any of these problems, it is important to consult your doctor.

I.

An Ancient Sleep

'. . . human vanity cherishes the absurd notion that our
species is the final goal of evolution'[1]

Richard Dawkins, *The Blind Watchmaker* (1986)

Sleep was a mystery to our distant ancestors. This is understandable. After all, until the nineteenth century, we knew very little about the brain. The sleep world you suddenly disappeared into every night had to be something supernatural. Some of this magic has disappeared with greater insight into the workings of our brain, but despite this, there are still many unanswered questions.

The way primordial humans slept may fit our current times better than you might expect. If we want to comprehend our own sleep, we need to look at the way our bodies have evolved over many thousands of years. Modern humans, *Homo sapiens*, evolved from older lineages between 230,000 and 300,000 years ago.[2]

That is very long ago, especially considering the fact that humans have only been living in cities for less than 10,000 years, that widespread use of electricity dates from the late nineteenth century, and that we have only had computers at home since the late 1970s.[3] Our brains have had to adapt very much to these developments in a relatively short time. Our living conditions have changed dramatically, but the evolution of our bodies and minds is not moving as fast.

In the field of sleep studies, learning from history is also interesting. Interpreting archaeological finds and observing contemporary hunter-gatherer societies helps us understand how primordial humans slept. Although details on the circadian rhythm (the physical, mental and behavioural changes an organism experiences over a 24-hour cycle) of our ancestors cannot be gleaned through archaeological findings, researchers have studied the lives of contemporary hunter-gatherers to get an idea of our day and night rhythms in the distant past. This has received some criticism, for example from Matthew Wolf-Meyer, anthropology professor at Rensselaer Polytechnic Institute, New York State. He states that because of modern social influences and other factors, no contemporary group can precisely be compared to people from an earlier evolutionary period.[4] On the other hand, in his 2010 monograph *The Hadza: hunter-gatherers of Tanzania*, Frank Marlowe, another professor of anthropology, while accepting that the Hadza are not 'living fossils', says it is amazing that they have preserved so much of their ancestral ways of life, with little changing since they were first officially described in 1911.[5]

The closest, therefore, we can get to getting a glimpse of sleep in the past is by studying a group with living conditions and a lifestyle that is far less influenced by modern-day technology, artificial lighting, and temperature regulation than our own. These circumstances are much more comparable to those in which primordial humans lived.

Bunk beds

The prehistoric period, by definition, is the period from which no 'legible' written sources exist. In other words, the historical record seems as illegible as my own prehistoric handwriting. The prehistoric period began 3–5 million years ago and ended around 3300 BCE. When you think of that period, an image of a cave dweller may come to mind – a man holding a club in his hand, trying to fend off a sabre-toothed tiger. At least, that is the first thing that comes to my mind. When I see pictures of a prehistoric human, I always get the feeling that the artist must have hated prehistoric people and thought little of their intelligence. The cave dwellers often look somewhat silly, making it almost impossible to imagine that they discovered fire or invented the wheel. I personally think primal humans were much smarter than these depictions.

Primal humans lived as hunter-gatherers, usually travelling from place to place. They lived in groups and hunted wild animals. They also collected things like nuts, seeds, plants, material for clothing, and wood for making fires. Today you go to the store for vegetables or a piece of meat, and on a lazy day you can have a ready-made meal delivered to your home. In prehistoric times, people of course had no access to such luxuries. After a day of hunting and gathering, it was important to rest well.

So, what did the 'bedroom' look like in prehistoric times? Although primordial man slept on the ground, it was not always that way. Their ancestors resided in nests in trees. There was an obvious reason for this. High up in the trees, they were protected from predators.[6] One sleep phenomenon in modern man may be a relic of those times. You may recognise it: you are nodding off and suddenly you are jolted awake with a falling sensation. Immediately you are awake! Pretty embarrassing when you are in class, an important but boring meeting, or on the train. We also call those muscle contractions hypnic jerks. Why does this phenomenon occur? It was probably important for survival. After all, if you are a tree-nesting inhabitant who falls asleep in an unfavourable place at high altitude, you could easily drop out of a jungle tree. As your body's muscles contract for a moment, you are startled awake and are able to check that you are in a safe place.

From the time primitive humans started using fire, it became less necessary to spend our nights in trees, as lighting campfires at night kept predators at bay. There was a significant advantage to sleeping on the ground. Primal man got a more stable night's rest than in the dangerous heights, which probably led to deeper and less interrupted slumber. That improvement had a positive effect on the brain in general. Our current cognitive intelligence might even be the result of the transition from tree sleep to ground sleep.[7]

The earliest bed that has been discovered dates from around 200,000 years ago. What did it look like? Well, it was of course not a box spring with padded headboard and lovely quilt. It was rather less comfortable and consisted of grass, branches and leaves, and it was located in a cave.[8] You might think that such a place was no fun to doze off in at all, but there is more. Next to the influence of changing weather circumstances, strong variations in temperature and the possible presence of dangers, insects terrorised primal man at night. How do we know? Insect-repellent plants covered the prehistoric bed! If you are an artist who portrays our primeval relatives, if you happen to read this, and if you then decide to draw a primeval man with a silly look in his eyes, I demand that you erase your drawing immediately! They were actually very resourceful types, our ancestors. That insecticide, by the way, was not the only extraordinary finding. Archaeologists found ashes in the various layers of the bed. Primal humans had rather unconventional methods of changing their beds and chasing away insects. They regularly set fire to their beds after sleeping on them. This probably had an effect not only on the creatures that were already crawling around in their bed, but also on any new intruders. Most crawling insects cannot move properly through fine powder because it blocks their breathing and causes dehydration.[9] (I can totally see how the bed-burning ritual would translate to our present day. Imagine if everyone set fire to their bed after sleeping in it once. Then every morning you'd be standing with your trailer at the dump with rows of cars behind you.

It's a good thing we have other ways of changing our beds these days. We have washing machines now and our beds thankfully no longer smell of burnt branches, but of wild honey or fresh lavender.)

Interestingly, primal humans also had other uses for their beds than dozing off on them. The bed was also a workplace for manufacturing stone tools used for hunting, for cleaning animal hides, and for food preparation. We can deduce this from stone shards found at the sleeping place.[10] Imagine sawing through a series of wooden planks on a newly made bed and then trying to fall asleep in between the sawdust and tools. Say goodbye to a nice night's rest! In addition to stone shards, grains of red and orange ochre covered the beds. Primal man probably used these for decorating their bodies or for colouring objects.

Did cave dwellers simply have sex in their beds? We do not know exactly, but to answer these questions, researchers have studied the habits of modern hunter-gatherers, whose living conditions have remained pretty much the same for thousands of years. The Aka tribe was one of the groups in which sexual activity was examined. They live in the tropical forest region of the Central African Republic. The Aka are primarily net-hunting foragers who don't live in caves, but in camps on the ground. The studies show that while some men are polygamous, the vast majority are monogamous.[11] Because in modern hunter-gatherers polygamy is only seen in a very small part of the population, it is likely that sex in prehistoric peoples was between two steady partners.[12]

Sexual activity in most tribes, such as the Aka, is typically covert. This means that the place where people sleep in groups is not the same as the place where they would have sex, because other tribe members would see the lovers in the act. For example, some of the Aka foragers in the study explained that they had sex in the forest, away from the rest of the tribe, while others had sex in their huts.[13] A reason for not having sex in the open might be to reduce shame, but also jealousy and mating competition.[14] From research into contemporary tribes such as the Aka, we might conclude that prehistoric peoples used their beds for rest and for work but less commonly for sex. As I will discuss in Chapter 6, sexual activity generally enhances sleep, so possibly they went to their beds quickly after the act to still benefit from its positive soporific effects.

Sleep, eat, move, repeat

Prehistoric man is regularly an inspiration for new insights into health and wellness. One well-known example is the 'Paleolithic diet'. Primal man is thought to have lived on a range of meat, fish, vegetables, fruits and nuts; according to the adherents of the Paleo diet, these are still the best sources of nutrition for modern man. There are, of course, proponents and opponents, but there is evidence that certain tenets of the Paleo diet constitute sound nutritional advice.[15] How did this primordial diet influence sleep?

Hundreds of thousands of years ago, humans learned how to cook with fire. They began to use stone tools for different purposes and to access food more easily. Researchers such as anthropologist Katharine Milton suggest that primitive man ate both vegetables and meat; others claim that more vegetables were eaten than lean meat, and others that fish was the most important staple.[16,17] Modern hunter-gatherer tribes now generally eat around 30 per cent animal-based food and 70 per cent vegetables (in extremely cold areas, such as the Arctic, however, they feed almost exclusively on animals).[18]

Around 10,000 years ago, our diet started to change. It was the beginning of the agricultural era and people began to eat more grains, legumes, dairy products and vegetable oils. In the modern era, another big transition to other food resources occurred. The industrial period that started around 1760 brought in more efficient farming methods, increased access to certain food sources, and ultimately opened the way to new food preservation techniques, with products such as canned meats, condensed soup and white bread becoming available.[19]

In 2003, anthropologist Clark Spencer Larsen from the Ohio State University in Columbus claimed that the transition from our Paleolithic diet to the diet of the agricultural era led to a mismatch between our bodies' needs and the type of food we ate. Evidence for this hypothesis comes from research that suggests that hunter-gatherers had a lower risk of age-related and chronic disease than agricultural workers. Possibly this has to do with the fact that people in the agricultural period started to eat a smaller range of food types, which contained fewer absorbable nutrients.[20]

Critics state that this effect had more to do with the fact that prehistoric hunter-gatherers perished early, so they did not reach an age in which chronic disease would develop.[21] Evidence for the exact state of health of prehistoric humans is scarce. However, we can compare modern hunter-gatherers with people from industrialised societies. Research shows that when comparing young hunter-gatherers with young people from industrialised countries, the former show lower rates of obesity, hypertension and insulin resistance. It might have to do with the combination of food that is more compatible with our Paleolithic DNA but also with the hunter-gatherers' activity levels, which are often much higher than those of populations in industrialised societies.[22]

So, if there were health benefits of the Paleolithic diet, how could it have influenced the way people sleep? One of the characteristics of the diet is that it is high in protein, which might have had a positive influence on the cave dwellers' night's rest. More specifically, high-protein meals such as in the Paleo diet show good effects on sleep, while poor sleepers get their energy more from carbohydrates and fats.[23] In addition, the original Paleolithic diet contained relatively few sugars, and scientific research shows that low-sugar diets might still have a positive effect on sleep in modern humans.[24] At the end of Chapter 5, I will elaborate further on the characteristics of the Paleolithic diet that might have promoted a good night's rest.

Contemporary hunter-gatherers have a very different activity pattern compared to people in industrialised societies: on average, males take between 18–19,000 steps per day and females around 11,000 steps. In contrast, in the United States, the average adult takes around 5,000 steps per day – a big difference from how it used to be.[25]

From this, we might conclude that primordial man was way more active than we are nowadays, which must have had a positive effect on overall health and sleep. Research suggests that low levels of physical activity are another evolutionary mismatch: in other words, we are moving too little to stay healthy, but that is not completely new! In 2021, Daniel Lieberman and colleagues stated that people who were more active in the prehistoric age survived better through the evolutional process of natural selection because they were better able to provide for and take care of offspring. This in turn led to the selection of people who were better able to repair and maintain the body after physical activity, which might have decreased their risk of chronic disease. The 'active grandparent hypothesis' is another term for this theory. Put differently, trying to find more food led to more exercise, which led to greater need for recovery, which promoted sleep.[26]

Nowadays access to food is easy for most people and we have all the resources within reach. The result is that there is less need for physical activity for direct survival, leading to an increase of inactivity. This inactivity can result in less need for recovery and for sleep. Our current lifestyles probably do not promote health and sleep as much as those we once had.

In short, living in the prehistoric age was probably more in line with the health needs and sleep needs of our bodies. Cave dwellers had to move more because they had to hunt for food and constantly find new food resources. Additionally, what they ate was better for sleep than many of the processed and sugar-rich foods we eat nowadays.

This almost sounds as if we all have to live like cave dwellers again because they had such positive health-promoting behaviour. However, research shows that they sometimes also indulged in unhealthy behaviours. I was quite surprised to find that they drank alcohol, and used nicotine and other stimulants. The earliest evidence of the use of nicotine dates from more than 12,000 years ago. Excavations at the Wishbone site in Salt Lake Desert in Utah exposed charred seeds of a tobacco plant in a small fireplace. It is unclear exactly how the hunter-gatherers used the plant material. Perhaps they smoked tobacco, but it might also be that they chewed it then spat it out.[27] It seems that the cave dwellers also drank a kind of primordial wine. Cave archaeologists found alcohol in storage jars in an excavation site in China. In Henan province, a beverage of rice, honey and fruit dates from 7,000 BCE. These drinks were likely of social, religious and medical significance.[28]

A few millennia later, around 5,000 years ago, there was already beer in China. Archaeologists analysing pottery vessels found evidence of ingredients such as barley and broomcorn millet.[29] This indicates that the people of ancient China not only brewed beer, but also used specialised tools for the task. In addition, research shows that cave dwellers would have sometimes been high on drugs. Analysis of Bronze Age human hair found on the island of Menorca shows that they used the alkaloids ephedrine, atropine and scopolamine. These psychoactive substances can induce realistic hallucinations, disorientation and alteration of sensorial perception, and were probably used to help people reach other states of mind, connecting them differently or more intensely to nature, each other, or gods in ritual ceremonies.[30]

I must say my image of cave dwellers changed a little after examining this research; somehow it was a relief that they might have not been that different from modern humans after all. Of course, the use of alcohol, alkaloid-bearing plants and nicotine would not have been very sleep-promoting, but they must have had many other things on their minds than trying to sleep well – maybe they did not even really try, because probably lying awake was not really something to worry about. In Chapter 4, I will examine the fact that modern hunter-gatherers do not even have a word for bad sleep, because they usually do not perceive a sleep problem as we would.

Better safe than sorry

The location of archaeological findings gives us information about the probable lifestyle of our ancestors. Based on this, we can conclude that the night was a dangerous period and that primal man sometimes had to make difficult choices between sleeping and staying awake.

Many of our modern sleep problems likely have their origins in prehistoric times, when it was vital to have a good balance between adequate slumber and sufficient alertness.[31] At night, primeval humans were probably easy prey for predators: this must have had an effect on their night's rest. Why risk sleep when danger could strike at any moment? I can imagine that you do not doze off well if a sabre-toothed tiger could be next to your bed at any moment. I would have sneakers ready on either side of the bed to make a good dash, since I do not think the chances of surviving a stare-down are high.

Individual sleep differences were probably very important for the safety of the tribe.[32] When you doze off, you are quite vulnerable to danger because you have less perception of your surroundings. As a result, you react more slowly to threats. In 1966 psychologist Frederik Snyder postulated his 'sentinel hypothesis' in which he stated that man and other animals stayed safe during sleep only if certain groupmates remained vigilant.[33]

As you can imagine, it made sense for prehistoric humans to do many daily activities together with others, but also to share their nights and to sleep in groups. That way, they were more likely to have someone alert when actual danger was at hand. Light sleepers were more alert at night, and early and late sleepers ensured that not everyone was in a deep slumber at the same time if predators or hostile tribes beset the group. Primal man probably slept a lot more soundly if he knew that an easily startled fellow tribesman was watching over him. In Western countries, it is almost impossible to imagine sleeping in large groups. The few times I spent the night in a dorm room as an adult during outings with friends felt a bit like a punishment. One after another was snoring or moving during the night and I noticed that it was not helping my sleep. I guess it's just what you're used to. Maybe I would sleep better in a group if I had learned to do so as a child.

It is of course impossible to test the sentinel hypothesis of sleep in prehistoric man. However, we can look at the behaviour of contemporary hunter-gatherers who are more subject to natural influences than industrialised societies. For example, the sleep of certain adult tribe members from Tanzania, Bolivia and Namibia has been examined using actigraphy.[34] This method, which measures physical activity levels using wristwatch-like motion detectors, is quite accurate in making a distinction between sleep and wake in average sleepers.[35] Evolutionary anthropologist Professor David Samson and research colleagues used this method to study the Hadza in Tanzania.[36] They live in an environment with a mean temperature of 17 degrees Celsius (63 degrees Fahrenheit) and their territory is primarily savanna woodland. People often move in and out of their groups, which comprised approximately 25–30 individuals.[37] Males act primarily as hunters and females as primary gatherers.[38] Traditionally, the Hadza used skinned animal hides as mattresses. Though some still do so, nowadays they most often use bedding materials such as textile blankets and sheets and woven grass mats, obtained through trade.[39]

An interesting finding was that modern hunter-gatherers indeed showed great interpersonal variation in their sleep schedules. Age was an important factor related to these differences. Older participants in the study tended to go to bed earlier, have more frequently interrupted sleep and wake up earlier than the younger ones. This led Samson and his colleagues to their 'poorly sleeping grandparent hypothesis'. This refers to the idea that older people, who went to sleep earlier and often woke up in the middle of the night, might have helped the tribe to survive because they could keep watch during the night and early mornings.[40]

The fact that older people wake up earlier also fits with my own experience. My grandfather and grandmother, with whom I lived as a child, were indeed up very early. I remember that my grandmother would start preparing the cooking upon rising, so that the whole house would smell of stew early in the morning. I didn't find that a problem, by the way. She could cook wonderfully. I can almost recall the smell just thinking about it!

The contemporary tribes as a whole had identical day–night rhythms. From this data, you might conclude that our sleep–wake (bio)rhythm is universal. Because the tribes people had no artificial light, temperature control or technological gadgets at their disposal, their natural environment primarily influenced their day–night rhythm. Thus, sleeping conditions were similar to those of primordial man.

I said that you might be able to conclude that our biorhythm was universal, except an actigraphy study in another pre-industrial society – that of an agricultural group living without electricity and technology in Madagascar – showed slightly different results. This has to do with the division of sleep into two phases. A common assumption is that primordial humans slept in two stages, with a long break in between in which they were awake. This two-phase idea relied on research by Roger Ekirch, professor of history, about sleep in the Middle Ages in Western Europe.[41] The belief was that we started sleeping differently after the industrial revolution and that continuous sleep suited us less. That change in sleep rhythm could explain insomnia. Yet the data from the sleep study of pre-industrial groups shows somewhat inconclusive results.[42,43]

In fact, hunter-gatherers did not sleep in two phases, while the Madagascar group did. More specifically, the average time of falling asleep of the Malagasy population was 7.21 p.m. and the average time of waking up was 5.44 a.m. After midnight, there was a strong increase of activity. This supports the notion of a biphasic sleep, as was normal in Western countries in the Middle Ages. In addition, the Malagasy showed napping in 88 per cent of the days and the average nap duration was a bit over 55 minutes.[44] In the Hadza tribe, sleep onset was much later, at 10.13 p.m. Their average time of waking up was over an hour later than the Malagasy, at 6.54 a.m., and they showed a more monophasic instead of segmented sleep. The Hadza napped on 54 per cent of the days and these naps lasted a little over 47 minutes.[45]

From these contradictory findings, you might conclude that our ancestors probably also showed major differences in their 24-hour rhythm. What could be the reason for these variations? Professor David Samson offered a potential explanation with his 'social sleep hypothesis'. He stated that humans are able to withdraw from the regular 24-hour cycle at any time and that this flexibility has helped us to survive. Sleeping in groups was one of the first adaptations: it enabled people to sleep in safer environments while others kept watch.[46] Just as it is for modern hunter-gatherers and the Malagasy, napping was probably a common occurrence in primordial humans, enabling them to recover physically and mentally in short periods. From this we can deduce that naps in the afternoon, such as during a siesta, must also have been a normal phenomenon in the past, with napping clearly longer than a power nap of 20–30 minutes. I will discuss this phenomenon further in Chapter 2.

This flexibility in sleep patterns most likely helped early humans to expand their habitat millions of years ago, when subgroups left Africa to travel to environments which had colder winters and stronger seasonal variations in terms of light exposure.[47] This must have been a challenge in terms of sleep. Not being able to sleep just anywhere because of the cold, and being dependent on fire and even more protected sleeping places may have led to different, more restricted sleeping patterns. The adaptability we show in terms of sleep probably helped us with this. People moved from camp to camp and the colder the days became, the more they became dependent on warmth from fire and warm clothing. The places where they could sleep were more limited. If you can no longer sleep just anywhere, it's probably better to compress your total bed time (the total time spent in bed). In addition, in countries far from the Equator, light exposure can differ greatly in winter and summer, which can lead to pitch-black days or white nights. That also probably contributed to the fact that we could no longer easily sleep all the time. The adaptability of our sleep system has therefore likely been essential for survival in environments other than the equatorial regions of Africa.

Samson found that a significant difference between the pre-industrialised groups and a Western population was that the first group showed a more consistent circadian rhythm, with fewer fragmented periods of rest and activity. This probably has to do with a greater influence of robust natural factors such as light and temperature on our sleep.[48] Nowadays we can influence these factors ourselves by using, for instance, air conditioners and lamps, which means that there can be greater differences in these circumstances between days. In Chapter 3, I will elaborate more on the influence of light and temperature on our biological clock and sleep quality.

Another important finding by evolutionary ecologist and anthropologist Gandhi Yetish was that the modern hunter-gatherers slept an average of 5 hours and 42 minutes to 7 hours and 6 minutes per night.[49] It was striking that the Hadza, for example, slept for 6 hours and 15 minutes, while their total in bed time was approximately 9 hours and 10 minutes. The Hadza were awake for an average of 22 minutes before falling asleep. At night, they were awake for almost 2½ hours. Despite this, they did not see being awake at night as a problem. It is of course true that traditional tribes nap more often, which can lead to more sleep than the above range. However, research among the Hadza showed that because napping did not occur every day, it only provided an average of about 17 minutes of extra sleep per day. This resulted in a total sleep of just over 6½ hours per 24 hours.[50]

Most people in industrialised countries would consider such a sleeping pattern to be terrible, but the Hadza don't seem to worry about lying awake at night. They just sleep, or they don't. In retrospect, when I suffered from insomnia, I often had a pattern like that of the Hadza. I kept relatively long total bed times just to get more sleep and then lay awake more and longer. An important difference was that I often worried while lying awake, especially about sleep itself and not getting enough shut-eye. You can imagine that a night worrying takes a lot more energy than if you just lie awake relaxed. More on this later.

From research on sleep in modern hunter-gatherers, we might deduce that our ancestors often had less than 8 hours of shut-eye. Now, the question is: where did the modern 8-hour advice come from? The industrial revolution in the late eighteenth and early nineteenth centuries played an important role. At that time, new norms and values emerged, resulting in a structured workday comprising longer working hours. The use of gaslights in streets stretched the hours of daytime and increasingly dispelled nights. People often worked 10–16 hours a day, 6 days a week. Robert Owen, a manufacturer turned social reformer from Wales, rebelled against these long working hours, creating the campaign slogan: '8 hours labour, 8 hours recreation, 8 hours rest'.[51]

Primal man, who lived hundreds of thousands of years before, did not follow that kind of rigid routine. He probably was able to find a good balance between sleep and the challenges presented by the natural environment. Campaigns such as Owen's, for factory workers doing long shifts to get much-needed rest and recuperation, placed a focus on balancing work and rest. From a sleep therapy perspective, this concept can lead to high expectations around getting a good night's rest, which can lead to even more sleep problems. As a therapist, I often saw this in practice. That golden rule of 8 hours seemed so ingrained in people. I will explain the sense and nonsense of this rule in more detail later in this book.

An assumption often made by sleep experts is that ambient light primarily influenced primordial man's circadian rhythms. According to this, primal man got up when it got light and went to bed when it got dark. There is now evidence that this was not quite the case. In fact, decreases and increases in ambient temperature also strongly influence our circadian rhythm. Modern hunter-gatherers get up some time before sunrise and go to bed a few hours after sunset. In one study, when temperatures dropped, the participating tribes went to bed, and when it got warmer, they got up.[52] Next time you turn the heating up in the evening, you might want to reconsider. After all, the question is whether it fits well with our biological clock. I will tell you more about that in the next chapter.

2.

What is Sleep?

'Nothing is as natural to us as sleep'[1]

Emanuel Wertheimer, *Aphorisms* (1897)

Cave dwellers may or may not have thought about why we doze off, but they might also have had interesting theories. We will never know exactly how they looked upon a night's rest. In the past decades, we have learned more and more about this interesting process that covers almost one-third of our lives. Well, as I will discuss later, for some it is one-third and for many readers a quarter, which is not necessarily a problem.

Sleep is a reversible and repetitive state of lowered consciousness. When you sleep you notice far less of what is going on around you and can react less adequately and quickly. Unlike drunkenly wandering the streets every weekend and dropping your keys in a gutter for the umpteenth time, this is a natural biological process. During this period, you partially shut yourself off from outside stimuli, but you also remain partially alert, and that is a good thing. After all, if this were not the case, you would be in danger every time you slept. For example, suppose your house catches fire at night: you must be able to react, despite the fact that you're asleep. The consequences would otherwise be disastrous. This is one of the reasons why many people refrain from using earplugs. They are afraid to be late for work or anxious about the idea that they might not hear that night-time intruder. I don't have much anxiety about sleeping through unsafe situations. I have been wearing earplugs every night since I was twenty-five. That habit started when I lived in an apartment above a supermarket, and early every Sunday a large truck unloaded food. After a night out, I wasn't expecting a loud beeping noise at 7 in the morning. I now use them every day. If I sleep somewhere else and don't happen to have them with me, I can sometimes look forward with suspense to trying to sleep without earplugs. Perhaps that is still a remnant of the period when I suffered from insomnia myself.

There are two main theories about why we sleep. The adaptive theory states that animals sleep to avoid danger from predators during a period in which, for most diurnal species, they can rely less on their sense of sight.[2] This theory explains why an animal would hide through the night, but not why it sleeps. On the other hand, it might be plausible that an animal would best conserve energy in a period in which it is less able to rely on vision and is not foraging for food. Another theory, the restorative theory, describes how sleep serves different functions. According to this theory, it helps with rest and repair, detoxifies, and enhances the immune response and learning.[3] Indeed, research shows that these functions increase during slumber in some animals. Possibly a combination of both theories provides the best explanation: being adaptive to the environment *and* making room for specific restorative functions are important reasons why we sleep.

In the animal kingdom, the duration of sleep and wakefulness varies greatly. In most animals, the active period is geared to the availability of prey, the threat of predators and opportunities for reproduction. For example, it is more advantageous for a lion to hunt at night. His night vision gives him the edge over animals that are less able to orient themselves in the dark. During the day, it is too hot to hunt, and so he takes that time to nap in the shade. I keep saying he, but of course, I should mostly say she, because the lionesses take care of 90 per cent of the pride's hunting. They are beautiful beasts, those male lions, but they are also huge sloths.

We still know relatively little about animal sleep. Indeed, we have only studied a fraction of the estimated 7.7 million animal species left on our planet.[4] Remarkably, a number of studies have concluded that some animals seem to have *no* fixed recurring period of lowered consciousness at all, which might mean that they do not sleep.[5] One such species often mentioned is the bullfrog. In a 1967 study, researcher J. A. Hobson delivered electrical shocks to several bullfrogs in the beginning and middle of the rest period and found that they had a stronger respiratory response later at night.[6] Hobson concluded that the animal reacted more during deep rest and concluded that this must be proof of an absence of sleep. However, later scientists discovered that in many species (including *Homo sapiens*), most deep sleep occurs at the beginning of the night, which suggests that the opposite is true, and that the bullfrog does indeed sleep![7]

Another species in which scientists have questioned the presence of sleep is the dolphin, because it moves continuously. However, research shows that it has the magical capability to only allow one half of its brain to sleep at a time, also called unihemispheric sleep.[8] In conclusion, we cannot be certain of the existence of an animal that does not sleep, but what we can conclude is that sleep (when present) comes in all shapes and sizes.

When you compare the sleep of humans with that of other primates, there are several specific differences. First, we are one of the few species who are habitual ground sleepers. Only male chimpanzees and male gorillas, who have few natural predators, also sleep on the ground.[9]

Second, we are extreme short sleepers. Scientists have tried to model human sleep duration by comparing it to that of other primates, based on factors such as body mass, brain size and diet. According to the model, we should sleep an average of 9½ hours, and not the 7 hours we habitually do. Third, we have a very high proportion of REM sleep (or dream sleep). Why we have such short sleep may be due to the evolutionary importance of long sleep duration compared to other behaviours. For example, Charles Nunn and his colleagues describe that, from an evolutionary perspective, an animal can sleep for a shorter amount of time if matters such as mating, searching for food or protection against predators become more important.[10] The latter is of course very important for *Homo sapiens*, given that by sleeping on the ground we became more vulnerable to predators.[11]

Stages

You might consider sleep as a state in which your body shuts down, like a TV on standby. One minute you can watch a movie and the next all you see is a little red light. Waking up is equivalent to pressing the power button on your remote control: in a flash, the screen is back.

However, the reality is a little different. In fact, your body is quite active during sleep. You go through several alternating sleep stages during the night. You can compare this process to going up and down stairs between an attic of being fully awake and a basement of deep sleep. You start at the top of the stairs and go a good number of steps into the dark depths of a deep slumber. Then you return to a place near the top of the stairs and then go back into the depths again. This process repeats itself about three times, but your sleep is not yet over. In fact, you go back to near the top of the stairs a few more times consecutively, only to go up and down a few steps. So deep sleep, also called NREM3 (stage 3 Non-rapid eye movement) occurs mainly at the beginning of the night, during the first 4½–5 hours after dozing off. Towards the end of the night, you mainly have light sleep (NREM1 and 2) and dream sleep (REM). A sleep cycle is a pattern in which different stages alternate before you return to NREM1 (or awake) and go back into a new one. During the night, an adult goes through 4–6 cycles, with an average length of 96 minutes per cycle in adults.[12] It is often suggested that all adults have average cycles lasting 90 minutes, and that the optimal time to wake up is after 6 hours or 7½ hours because then you are sure to wake up at the end of a 90-minute cycle. This should promote a more refreshed feeling in the morning. However, the duration of cycles varies between people. In some adults, an average cycle lasts a mere 60 minutes, while in others, it can even last 150 minutes or longer. Evidence suggests that genetic variation is the main reason for these differences.[13] I've never had sleep studies done on myself, so I wouldn't know how long my sleep cycles last.

I often notice that I wake up around 6.30 a.m. when I go to bed at midnight. Usually, I need the first half hour to wake up, but then I can start my day fresh. That was different during my period of insomnia. At that time, I would get out of bed very tired in the morning and the tiredness would last all day. I often also saw that pattern in my patients. Waking up itself was often not a problem as a patient with insomnia, but a lack of energy sometimes prevented me from getting out of bed. A phase of sleep in which waking up is often very difficult is deep sleep. Have you ever tried to wake someone in the first hours after falling asleep? That can be quite a challenge. Even a glass of water in the face cannot wake some at such a time (don't try this at home). On the contrary, a small sound might startle someone who is in NREM1 or NREM2. For example, think back to when as a teenager you came home from a party excessively late and did not want to wake your parents. Even though you tried so hard to sneak up the stairs, they were awake because of that one creaking step. A piece of advice for adolescents is that it is best to come home late within the first 4½–5 hours of your parents' sleep, because if you want to sneak up the stairs later, you are more likely to find them in the light sleep stages and you are in for a problem.

We can investigate sleep by measuring brain activity, also known as brain waves. While you are reading this, your brain is producing about 16 brain waves per second. During NREM1 and NREM2, the brain is quite active, with brain waves being somewhat faster and more irregular. As you sink deeper into sleep, the waves become slower, deeper and more regular. During your dream sleep, a special phenomenon takes place. Your body is completely calm at that time, and you cannot use your muscles, but your brain waves are fast and irregular. You also see that people in this sleep stage show rapid eye movements. This is why another description for dream sleep is Rapid Eye Movement sleep, or REM sleep.

As our body develops from newborn to adult, our sleep changes as well. Specifically, this concerns the time spent in the different stages. In the first weeks of life, there is an even distribution of sleep and wakefulness across day and night, with no regular rhythm. Newborns spend up to 18 hours of the day sleeping. In contrast to children and adults, newborns start their cycle with active sleep (analogous to REM sleep) and each sleep contains one or two cycles. They have a great amount of REM sleep, adding up to 50 per cent of the total sleep time.[14] When the baby is 3 months old, sleep onset begins with NREM. At 6 months of age, babies sleep an average of 13 hours a day, over larger blocks of time.[15] Sleep amounts decrease when children get older. Total sleep time decreases from 13 hours to 11 hours between the ages of 2–5 years.[16] Most children discontinue napping between the ages of 3–5 years.[17] In adolescence, NREM3 and sleep latency time decreases, while time spent in NREM2 increases.[18] On average, an adult spends around 20–25 per cent in REM sleep and 20–25 per cent in NREM3. The rest is mostly NREM2, usually comprising 45–55 per cent of total sleep.[19]

The time of your life

In the eighteenth century, Jean-Jacques de Mairan demonstrated the existence of a physical clock that regulates our day–night rhythm. He was a French astronomer who placed a plant in a closet. The plant opened its leaves around the same time every day without the presence of sunlight.[20] Later, researchers discovered that many organisms, including animals and humans, have such a built-in biological clock.

Today, we are increasingly aware of how the biological clock affects our daily lives. You have probably experienced the following: during the working week, you get up at 7 a.m. every day. At the weekend, you go to bed a little later and you think: 'I'm going to get a good night's sleep by sleeping through the morning.' Alas! You wake up at 7 in the morning and find it hard to fall asleep again. Relatable? This is the influence of your biological clock. Many people have heard of this structure, but what is it exactly and where is it located in the body?

A main area that regulates our circadian rhythm is a brain structure called the suprachiasmatic nucleus (SCN), also known as the master clock. This structure is located in a part of the brain just above the junction of your optic nerves. That location is not a surprise. In fact, the amount of light reaching your retina affects the functioning of your biological clock.

Among other things, our biological clock regulates body temperature. During the day, our body temperature is higher than at night. At night the temperature gradually declines, which promotes the onset and maintenance of sleep. During the night, the body temperature drop can be 1 degree Celsius (about 2 degrees Fahrenheit). There is a gradual increase of body temperature again before waking up.[21]

Our biological clock appears to be discordant with the 24-hour rhythm of a day. We know this because of so-called cave experiments. During such an experiment, the subjects have no idea of time. In the cave, there is no light and the temperature is always the same. In these conditions, the biological clock exhibited a different rhythm than the 24-hour clock. In fact, our internal rhythm appears to restart on average after 24½ hours.[22] A salient detail surrounding these experiments is that one of the researchers himself participated as a test subject and spent 2 months in the dark environment. The things you do for science . . .

Probably you have heard of melatonin. The SCN controls the release of this hormone by the pineal gland. When it gets dark, it forces the pineal gland to release melatonin. Melatonin is a substance in the body that is involved in the timing of your sleep. Many people use melatonin in pill form to enhance sleep, but in reality there are only a few indications that it might have a positive effect on your sleep. (I will discuss this further in Chapter 10.) In addition to light, diet and exercise are also important factors that affect your biological clock. Additionally, as I described in the first chapter, ambient temperature is involved in regulating the day–night rhythm. Recent research findings in which the temperature of the environment had a direct influence on the functioning of the SCN support this.[23]

In short, the master clock is a busy little bee and a bossy little structure. It sometimes refuses to cooperate if you want to nap during the day. At that time, your body is not yet properly prepared for sleep, partially due to insufficient release of melatonin. This does not mean that you can never take a daytime nap. In fact, other factors play a role in being able to fall asleep, which I will come back to later.

As I wrote earlier, the day–night rhythm of hunter-gatherers is much more stable than that of people in industrialised countries. This has to do with the fact that their biological clock picks up many more direct environmental cues, such as light, that help to maintain a constant rhythm. You can imagine that a clearer signal of day or night is given if you get outdoor light all day and are gradually exposed to complete darkness in the evening. Of course, this cannot be compared to the poorly lit office spaces we stay in during the day and the brighter living areas in the evening. The cooler evenings due to the setting sun cannot be compared to the heated rooms we stay in at night. So, the difference between day and night is simply less clear to our biological clock. As we'll see in Chapter 5, variations in light and temperature still have a larger effect on sleep in contemporary hunter-gatherers than in people from industrialised societies. Climate control and artificial light might lead to smaller seasonal variations in sleep duration in the latter group.

East, west, home is best

If you have ever travelled east, you might recognise it: even after a long flight and a possibly energy-draining day travelling, you cannot manage to doze off at night. Tiredness and sleepiness during the following period might also be present. People experiencing these symptoms might think they are suffering from travel fatigue, but it usually has to do with the biological clock. Our body generally has more difficulty adjusting from a trip from west to east than vice versa. Since the biological clock inherently exceeds 24 hours, it is easier for our body to adapt to a longer than to a shorter day. The latter is the case when travelling to the east.

Even though your biological clock can adjust to the rhythm of a new time zone, it takes a while for it to do so. After all, your clock still ticks to the old time just after your trip. The greater the time difference between two zones, the longer it takes your clock to adjust to the new time zone. This phenomenon is also known as jet lag, and it may last anywhere from a few days to a few weeks.[24]

You can assume that for every hour your biological clock has to shift, you need one day to get into the new rhythm. This is true for a trip from west to east. A trip from east to west requires less adjustment time. You need one day to adapt for every 2-hour time shift when travelling west to get used to the new rhythm. So, if you are going from San Francisco to Amsterdam, then you need about 9 days for your body to get used to the new rhythm. If you are going from Amsterdam to San Francisco, you will need 4–5 days. In Chapter 10, I will describe effective strategies to combat jet lag.

Larks and night owls

You probably know a colleague who is always brimming with energy in the morning. It seems like he or she must have been awake for hours and must have had 3 cups of coffee. However, you know that person does not even drink coffee. If you are more of a morning person, that energy can be quite fun. If you are a genuine evening person and need just a little more time to get going in the morning, you may have a tougher time with that cheerful colleague in the early mornings.

I'm not really a morning person or a night person. I prefer to describe myself as an afternoon person. I get sleepy between 11 p.m. and 11.30 p.m. and wake up between 6.30 a.m. and 7 a.m. It means that I am not the most sparkling person in the morning because I often need another half-hour to wake up nicely, but it also means that I'm usually not the one who turns the lights off after a party. On average I'm quite happy with my rhythm. It kind of runs in my family. My parents both have a bit of the same rhythm and so does my older brother.

Your biological clock largely determines your circadian rhythm, and there are many individual differences. Some people's physical alarm clock goes off around 6 a.m., while others struggle to get out of bed by 9 a.m. or even 11 a.m. Although many might question these variations and put them down to signs of laziness in evening types, these variations are differences in *chronotype*, which have a biological basis. A chronotype refers to a person's natural inclination with regard to the times of day when they prefer to sleep or when they are most alert or energetic. On average, most people fall asleep between 11 p.m. and 12 midnight, but there are individual differences that appear to be especially genetically predisposed.[25] In the past, people were usually referred to as morning or evening types. However, this creates a notion of chronotype being a dichotomous characteristic, while it is not a matter of black and white but more of a spectrum, as with many individual traits involving the human body. This is why the concepts of 'morningness' and 'eveningness' were introduced in sleep science, with a person falling somewhere in between, either more towards the early or the later chronotype.

You are more likely to show morningness if one of your parents does as well. I saw this often in my work at the practice. Adolescents who have more trouble getting out of bed in the morning usually have one parent with the same problem. Besides genetics, age also plays an important role in how your biological clock works. In adolescents, there is usually a backwards shift of the clock, resulting in delayed sleepiness and more trouble getting out of bed early in the morning. On the contrary, as you get older, you seem to become more and more of a morning person. For example, it is normal to wake up on average at 7 a.m. at age 30 and at 6 a.m. at age 60. This is often a result of the influence of aging on our day–night rhythm. As discussed in Chapter 1, the reason why our biological clock changes throughout the years might have an evolutionary explanation. Variations in chronotype were a guarantee for people being wakeful at different points in the night, leading to greater protection from nocturnal dangers.

There also seems to be a clock difference between men and women.

Before the age of 40, women tend to show more morningness than men. Once over 40, men tend to become more early birds, while women remain stable in terms of the timing of their circadian rhythms.[26]

Another interesting factor is geographic location. People living further away from the Equator show more eveningness. An explanation for this might be that there are not only differences in light, but also in temperature when looking at latitude. However, in a large systematic review (a summary of available evidence from two or more separate studies) of over 35,000 people, it showed that sunset was the most important factor associated with the differences in eveningness and morningness.[27] This shows that next to temperature, light in the morning is essential for our sleep and circadian rhythm. In Chapter 5, I will address the exact influence of light on our sleep.

Midnight

We know that environmental factors are very powerful in determining our day–night rhythm, but behavioural factors are at least as important.

One behavioural factor is the siesta. The word means 'sixth hour' and indicates the time when people have a nap during the day and when shops close for a few hours in hot climates. The exact era in history that siestas became commonplace is difficult to pinpoint, although it is likely that they go back to at least Roman times. Nowadays the siesta is most often associated with Spain, although it is a tradition in other countries, including Greece and Central and South American countries. In Spain, a typical workday might run from 9 a.m. to 2 p.m., with a 2-hour break for the long nap, and work resuming at 4 p.m. and ending at 8 p.m. A 2016 Spanish study, however, found that siestas are no longer as popular in Spain as one might think. Almost 58 per cent of the Spanish surveyed never napped in the afternoon and only 18 per cent took a siesta four or more days in the week.[28] In Chapter 1, I suggested that siestas were probably an important part of life for prehistoric man, based on the fact that contemporary traditional peoples studied took a long afternoon nap on alternate days.

Our nights generally consist of a continuous period of sleep but, as noted earlier, according to Robert Ekirch this has not always been the case.[29] He stated that how people slept in much of Western Europe in the Middle Ages was very different to how it is now. Based on a combination of scientific, anthropological and textual evidence Ekirch concluded that sleep back then often consisted of two nightly parts: people usually had a first and second slumber and were awake for about an hour in between, also called biphasic sleep. Nowadays, it is not considered a positive thing if you spend an hour awake in the middle of the night, but research suggests that in the Middle Ages people actually saw this time as very beneficial. The first sleep took away most of the exhaustion and, in the quietness of the night, bedfellows could have casual conversations or sex without being disturbed. At the time, physicians even recommended having sex after the first sleep. After all, the doctors thought that this was a perfect opportunity to conceive children. Moreover, according to them, you could also get more pleasure from sex at that time.[30] In addition, people might use the hour to pray, or to do household chores. I think my neighbours would be very surprised to hear me vacuuming the floor in the middle of the night. However, if everybody's doing a big clean-up between 3 and 4 in the morning, it would seem less strange, of course. Recently, there has been criticism towards Ekirch's conclusions about biphasic sleep being a widespread common practice in the early Modern Period. In 2023, Niall Boyce, an English professor at the University of London, concluded that the evidence was ambiguous and he proposed a more diverse interpretation of early modern texts on sleep. For example, according to Boyce, the early references to 'first sleep' and 'second sleep' might represent different phases in a continuous sleep instead of two sleep phases separated by a long period of wake.[31]

As I described earlier, certain pre-industrial groups in Madagascar still have a sleep system in which they sleep in two parts. It seems as if there was no universal way of sleeping from an evolutionary point of view, because both biphasic sleep and single-period sleep occur in traditional peoples.

Under pressure

You may have experienced being in your car at night after a party, driving everyone back home. Some friends are snoring delightfully in the back seat after having one too many drinks. You try to focus on the dimly lit road ahead. Before you know it, you notice that your eyes are almost closing. In fact, you may well actually have dozed off for a microsecond. The phenomenon you are dealing with at that moment is sleep drive or sleep pressure.

The first description of the biological process of sleep pressure dates from the seventeenth century. The French philosopher René Descartes thought sleep had to do with a kind of pressure in our brain. He described how a substance he referred to as 'animal spirits' filled the brain's cavities, increasing the pressure in those cavities and allowing us to stay alert. According to Descartes, when the cavities were emptied, we fell asleep.[32] Researchers have long abandoned this theory, but we still talk about sleep pressure.

The higher your sleep pressure, the sooner you fall asleep. Think back to that class at school you tried to attend after a short night. Your neighbour might have briefly tapped you when your head was already on the table. Those are the effects of considerable sleep pressure.

While the hormone melatonin is very important for the regulation of the timing of sleep, adenosine is a neuromodulator responsible for the process of sleep pressure – the amount of sleepiness.[33] Adenosine is involved in storing and releasing energy throughout the body. When your body uses energy through muscle activity, it frees energy by using the compound adenosine triphosphate (ATP) and releases adenosine as a by-product. The brain is the part of the body that uses most ATP and, while doing this, it builds up adenosine in the space between the brain cells. This accumulation probably limits activity in certain parts of the brain, which causes decreased alertness.[34] It sounds like Descartes was not that wrong after all when he was talking about the animal spirits filling our brain during the day.

The longer you are out of bed and active, the higher your sleep pressure. So, if you are in bed too long, it can become more difficult to doze off at night, which can be annoying. For example, many people have difficulty falling asleep on Sunday nights. Often, they think it has to do with stress, and that they are too tense to sleep because they have to start the working week again.

This might be part of the explanation, but there is more. Normally there are between 16 and 17 hours between the time you get up and go to bed. This is why if you get out of bed at 11 a.m., you may not be sleepy enough in the evening. It is because your sleep pressure is too low. Therefore, the advice is that after that party until 3 in the morning, you should just get up at 8 a.m., put on your walking shoes and take a nice walk in the woods. Make sure you do not run into anyone and just go to bed at the normal time. If you still do not feel much enthusiasm for getting a breath of fresh air after 5 hours of sleep, try going to bed a little later on Sunday nights. Although your night is going to be a bit shorter than usual, your sleep pressure might now be high enough to fall asleep properly. As previously indicated, humans are the primates who sleep the least, and this may have to do with the fact that sleeping on the ground made us more vulnerable to predators. Building up sleep pressure ensures that we can sleep more efficiently in those short periods when confronted with danger.

In modern humans, we also see this principle reflected in sleep research. Shorter total bed times ensure that people experience relatively deeper sleep.[35] One of the most effective treatments for insomnia is building up sleep pressure, which significantly increases sleepiness and makes it easier to fall asleep and stay asleep. It was also one of the most important strategies that helped me improve my sleep. In Chapter 9, I will discuss this powerful treatment strategy in more detail.

A good team

To help our bodies keep a good 24-hour rhythm, the biological clock (often referred to as Process C) and sleep pressure (Process S) work together as the two main mechanisms controlling sleep and wakefulness. This means that at some times your sleep pressure might be high, but the time of day is off, which makes it more difficult to fall asleep. It also works the other way around, when the time of the day to go to sleep is fine, but you experience too little sleep pressure. The cooperation of our clock and sleep pressure is referred to as the two-process model of sleep–wake regulation.[36] It seems that the functioning of the biological clock decreases when sleep pressure is too high. This means that staying awake for too long makes you less sensitive to light and other cues to stay awake.[37]

This is what happens when you deprive yourself of sleep for too long. You will doze off no matter what the time of day is. I recognise this process when, for example, I get home late from a party. The next day I can sometimes just fall asleep on the couch in the evening.

Well, I should add that watching TV on the couch is definitely a sleep-inducing thing, for me anyway. I often resolve to watch a nice movie or interesting documentary, but might only see the beginning and the credits. This is not a good example of good sleep hygiene, but it shows that even as a sleep scientist you do not always follow the sleep rules perfectly.

Quality time

How do you know if your sleep is of good quality? Sleep quality is a broad concept and can mean different things depending on how it is measured. There is a difference between subjective and objective sleep quality. Subjective sleep quality refers to how you experience your sleep and is measured by questionnaires or a sleep log (which I will discuss further in Chapter 9). Questionnaires can specifically measure insomnia or symptoms related to medical conditions such as sleep apnoea, in which a person's breathing is disrupted while they sleep. The most common form is obstructive sleep apnoea (OSA), which is a sleep disorder in which obstruction of the upper airway occurs. This leads to a loss of oxygen in the blood and may have many negative consequences for cardiovascular health.[38]

The difficulty with some of the most commonly used questionnaires in research, such as the Pittsburgh Sleep Quality Index (PSQI), is that the total score does not give an indication of the type of sleep complaint.[39] Many scientists only use this total score when presenting their research data. This often makes a statement like 'cardiovascular problems are associated with poor sleep quality' difficult to interpret. Are the researchers addressing subjective sleep problems in initiating or maintaining sleep, or do they refer to symptoms caused by a medical condition such as OSA? In Chapter 3, I will discuss what the consequences are of this lack of clarity for the interpretation of research surrounding health and sleep. I addition, I will explain why this can lead to unnecessary worry and anxiety for people who suffer from insomnia.

Is your daytime energy level a good determinant of the quality of your sleep? Not necessarily! Fatigue can be caused by many factors, including insomnia. However, not all fatigue has to be directly related to your sleep. To map subjective sleep quality, it is not only important to look at daytime fatigue, but also at your experience of how long it took to fall asleep and how long and often you were awake at night.[40] By the way, it is often even more important to look at the way you felt and how stressed you were while awake. More about that shortly.

The experience of sleeping or waking is a very interesting phenomenon, and it seems that our brains trick us sometimes. For example, half of good sleepers perceive a sleep state only after they have objectively slept for 22 minutes without disturbance. Moreover, people with insomnia need 34 minutes of objective undisturbed sleep to experience that they have actually slept.[41] Apparently, we do not observe periods of shorter and interrupted naps as sleep. This probably partly explains why people with insomnia often greatly underestimate their total sleep duration. They sometimes think they have slept hours less than measured in a sleep study. Because of the fragmentation of their night's rest, they often experience sleep as wakefulness.

In practice this might mean that sleep duration is good in most people with insomnia, but the fragmentation leads them to underestimate it. Therefore, increasing the subjective sleep quality and enhancing the experience of sleep is one of the most important goals of treatment.

When I discuss subjective sleep quality, I am also referring to the way you view lying awake. In Chapter 1, I described how the Hadza showed sleep patterns that for many people would be a sign of very poor sleep. In fact, their sleep doesn't even come close to what Western people consider good subjective sleep quality. In think the reason why we value continuous sleeping probably has to do with the way many of us lie awake when we can't sleep. It is more natural for the Hadza to be disturbed by their bedmates at night, since the entire family is in one bed. For us solitary sleepers, this is unimaginable. It is simply less normal for us to lie awake because we usually have less external disturbance. If we then start worrying about it, the circle is of course complete. The Hadza simply have more 'restful wake', which is a term I will use frequently throughout this book. This means that their nocturnal waking moments are probably relaxing. In contrast, because of stress and rumination, these periods are energy-consuming periods for us and this itself might lead to a more negative experience of the night.

Another difference between the Hadza and people from industrialised countries is that, according to actigraphy, we generally have shorter total bed times. On average, the Hadza adults are in the bed for just over 9 hours, while we have a total bed time of around 8 hours. Nevertheless, we have the same amount of sleep as the Hadza. We sleep an average of around 6 hours and 10 minutes, which is similar to the 6 hours and 15 minutes of the Hadza.[42] This means that people from industrialised countries probably build up more sleep pressure, which generally leads to less fragmented sleep. Our definition of a good sleeper has changed accordingly. In other words, we have probably forgotten how to lie awake at night and have learned to see this as a problem. My theory is that this has created mental pressure for many around the need to sleep continuously and it is one of the reasons why industrialised societies often glorify uninterrupted sleep. Accordingly, many of my patients viewed continuous sleep as a personal achievement. This association with achievement hardly occurs naturally in contemporary hunter-gatherers, which was likely also the case in primordial humans.

As a sleep therapist, my experience of people with insomnia is that this mental pressure leads to longer and more stressful waking periods. As I will describe in Chapter 9, the solution for people with insomnia is often not to simply lie in bed longer, because that would prolong the already stressful waking moments. Rather, it is about shortening the stressful waking moments so that the individual regains a restful period during the night. So, if you are unable to create relaxed wake periods, it is better to have as little wakefulness as possible during the night.

Next to reporting subjective sleep quality, it is also possible to measure sleep quality in an objective way. This can be done by using commercial sleep technologies such as smartwatches, but also by using professional instruments. There are specific disorders that, while the perception of sleep might be fine, do negatively affect objective sleep quality. Examples of these are obstructive sleep apnoea or narcolepsy. In both these sleep disorders, there is a disruption of sleep which can result in excessive daytime sleepiness. Symptoms of obstructive sleep apnoea also include loud snoring and breathing stops during the night. Women with obstructive sleep apnoea are less likely to report snoring or sleepiness; they more often suffer from symptoms such as daytime fatigue, morning headaches and mood disturbances. In contrast with men, women more often show sub-jective insomnia symptoms and experience nightmares.[43] (To reiterate, if you experience excessive daytime sleepiness or if you show other symptoms of obstructive sleep apnoea, consult your doctor as a physical examination and/or a sleep study might be required.)

Which measuring approach is best for you depends on the type of sleeper you are, the symptoms you may have during the day or night and your specific need. If you are a good sleeper and want an indica-tion of your total bed time and insights into variations in sleep time and rhythm across time, a smartwatch can be the right instrument.[44] For people with insomnia, a smartwatch is much less reliable in measuring total sleep time,[45] and it is best to use measures of subject-ive sleep, such as a sleep log. In general, commercial sleep technology is not reliable when it comes to measuring sleep stages. Apps often measure your movement or your heart rate and sometimes give a somewhat elusive 'sleep score' that is probably not a good indication of your sleep quality. In my work, I have regularly encountered people who felt that they had slept well and only felt worse after receiving a low 'sleep score' on their smartphone. In Chapter 11, I will further discuss the sense and nonsense of commercial sleep measurements.

In people with daytime or night-time complaints that fit obstruct-ive sleep apnoea or other organic sleep disorders (such as daytime sleepiness or 'breathing stops' during the night), a doctor might refer the individual for polysomnography. Such a professional examin-ation comprises measurements of your brain activity, heart rate and a number of other physical factors to give an indication of the sleep phase you are in. You may think that such a sleep study will correlate well with how long and well you think you have slept, but that is not necessarily true. The scientific findings are mixed. According to a number of studies, lots of REM (dream) sleep, lots of deep sleep (NREM3), and less waking are linked to better subjective sleep quality.[46,47] Another large study, however, shows no correlations at all.[48] Subjective sleep quality is related to how you *feel*. The lower the subjective sleep quality, the more likely you are to be less optimistic, satisfied and positive during the next day.[49]

Researchers sometimes use objective measures such as polysom-nography to describe detailed variations in sleep structure and phases. They might use this to examine whether substance use or environ-mental factors can influence these objective sleep characteristics. Sometimes this type of research gives clues about what factors can hamper these aspects. In people with insomnia, polysomnography is usually not advised because the subjective experience is most important when assessing insomnia complaints and there is often a big discrepancy between the experience of insomnia complaints and the results of a polysomnography test. The same is true for actigraphy. Researchers often use it as an indication for sleep and wake, such as in the Hadza tribe. This method is quite accurate in measuring total sleep time when compared to polysomnography, especially in the general population.[50] In people with insomnia, an actigraphy over-estimates total sleep time (which I will discuss further in Chapter 9).[51]

In short, in most people, and especially in people with insomnia, the perception of your own sleep quality is associated more with day-time functioning than objective measurements. In the majority of cases, sleep studies provide little additional information, which is why the general advice is not to perform polysomnography tests on individuals who experience sleeplessness.

Later in this book I will summarise research on subjective as well as objective measurements of sleep. I will try to make a clear distinction between the two and place the scientific data within its context accordingly.

Just what you need

In the Middle Ages in Europe, sleeping in was considered unhealthy and a sign of laziness; this is still the case in many cultures.[52] Further-more, it was thought to induce headaches and fever. My clients often thought they needed 8 or even 9 hours of continuous slumber to counteract their fatigue. Do you need 8 hours? Some people do, but most do not. I usually compare optimal sleep duration with shoe size. If you walk in shoes that are too small or too big, you'll get blisters. In line with this, rest periods in bed that are too short or long can create more difficulty in daytime functioning. It is therefore important to find the right amount of sleep you personally need.

I discussed in the first chapter that the general advice of 8 hours has nothing to do with how we as humans probably naturally slept on average. If you sleep (much) less, I can imagine that the desire to sleep 8 hours can put quite a strain on you. This can lead to negative thoughts and feelings surrounding your sleep. Thoughts such as '7 hours of sleep is not enough' and 'if I don't get 8 hours of sleep, I will get sick and shorten my life' are counterproductive. In fact, the consequence of these beliefs is that people often try to sleep longer, which can lead to a decrease of adenosine and a decrease of sleepiness. In average sleepers this does not have to be a problem per se, because lying awake in itself is quite natural. However, in people with insomnia this can worsen sleeplessness, because the periods of restless wake are extended. As a former insomniac, I know what the pressure of the 8-hour rule can do to you. I would often look at the alarm clock at night to calculate how many hours of sleep I'd already managed and whether I would reach my goal of 8 hours. Because during that period I often felt like I didn't sleep more than 5 hours. I'd then get out of bed frustrated and dread the day ahead.

During my doctoral study, in which I examined more than 200 subjects, I found that insomniacs spend an average of 8½–9 hours in bed, just like I did during my bout of sleeplessness. This is more than a half-hour to an hour longer than average and for most people this leads to more restless wake.[53,54]

To recap, staying in bed longer than needed exacerbates the sleep problem because it reduces sleep pressure and increases periods of restless wake. If you have insomnia this can end up in a vicious circle. This is because those long total bed times cause you to have sleep that is more fragmented, which leads to more fretting about sleep. That in turn affects how you feel and how tense you are, which leads to problems with falling asleep, even more fragmented sleep and less restful night-time wake.

People with insomnia often think that average sleepers get 8 hours and that less is bad for you, which is not necessarily true: there are long and short sleepers. Moreover, 8 hours is much higher than the general average. In fact, about 60 per cent of the population over the age of 18 subjectively sleep 7 hours or less, and nearly 30 per cent report sleeping 6 hours or less.[55] For many people who thought getting 8 hours of sleep was a necessity, this might be quite a relief.

Sleeping less than 8 hours is usually not a problem at all. In 2015, a team of experts at the US National Sleep Foundation downgraded the required sleep duration for adults, concluding that 6 hours of sleep can also be sufficient.[56] As long as you function well, you can often get by just fine with less sleep. For people with insomnia, focusing on the subjective quality of sleep first is usually more important. I will tell you more about this in Chapter 9.

In the past, many researchers have expressed assumptions around sleep duration that were not supported by scientific literature and were not helpful for people with insomnia. They suggested that adults from industrialised countries are increasingly suffering from a massive sleep deprivation epidemic because they give themselves too little time to sleep, and that this epidemic has terrible health consequences. In recent years, research has shown that these horror stories are incorrect. An extensive review from 2017 describes that in adults, there is little evidence supporting this assertion.[57] Instead, they found that objective sleep time had not declined over a period of fifty years. However, they did describe that subjective sleep quality has decreased since the 1990s. It is not sleep quantity but *subjective sleep quality* that is becoming the bigger problem. In my opinion, creating absurd standards of sleep duration only worsens the problem because people who sleep badly get frustrated and anxious if they don't achieve the idealised 8 hours.

Nevertheless, this does not mean that there is no group that has slept less over time. In 2015, Katherine Keyes and research colleagues mentioned adolescents as a group that requires attention when it comes to sufficient sleep. Between 1991 and 2012, the percentage of US adolescents who reported sleeping less than 7 hours increased by 30 per cent.[58] Among other factors, Keyes et al. suggested that social media and increasing demands of school and extracurricular activities might explain the trend of less sleep in adolescents.

A common misperception is that sleeping longer is the primary means of combating fatigue. Why is this belief often incorrect? As I mentioned before, fatigue is a complex complaint with multiple causes. Often these are not (only) related to your night's rest. For example, too much physical and mental strain often leads to fatigue. If you are overworked, it can take a long time before you feel fit again. This then often has nothing to do with how long you slumber.

If fatigue is not a good indicator of your optimal sleep duration, how do you know how much you need? The answer to that question is not as straightforward as one might expect. There are great individual differences in sleep needs.

One of the indicators of your optimal sleep duration is how sleepy you are during the day. Sleepiness is not the same as fatigue. Fatigue is about how much energy you have, while sleepiness is about the tendency to fall asleep (unwanted). For example, you may be very fit and enjoying the beach, but the heat and relaxation can make you sleepy and doze off despite your high energy level. In this case, you are not tired, but sleepy. It can also be the other way around. For example, you can be very tired after an afternoon of vigorous exercise, but when you lie down on the couch, you are still not sleepy enough to doze off.

Insomnia often has nothing to do with too little sleep but instead with poor sleep and less restful nocturnal wake. This is why, in people with insomnia, fatigue is often more prominent than sleepiness.[59] The fact that too little slumber is not the same as insomnia can be seen in people who have had too short total in-bed time over a long period; they have really little sleep. This causes them to fall asleep against their will during the day due to excessive sleep pressure, and we see this much less in insomniacs.[60]

In conclusion, daytime sleepiness is a good indication that you have not had enough of a night's rest. Sometimes the effects of a lack of sleep can be more subtle or even unnoticeable. If you are a good sleeper and you are not sure whether you are getting enough sleep, you might try extending your total bed times a bit and see whether you feel better after a couple of weeks. If this is the case and you are still experiencing good sleep at night, you might be on the right track by extending your total bed times.

For people with insomnia, not being sleepy at night is an indication that you should not focus on extending total bed times. Instead, shortening total bed times might lead to less fragmented sleep (and restless wake) because of an increase of sleep pressure. So, do you tend to lie in bed longer to get more night's rest, but spend much of that time lying awake (and being stressed)? Then you are probably expecting a longer sleep than you currently physically need. You are much better off focusing on getting good-quality night's rest first, and that means you may have to implement shorter total bed times. I will discuss ways to manage this in Chapter 9.

In the general population, it is more common to be a poor sleeper than a short sleeper. A recent study showed that 22 per cent of people suffer from insomnia, while approximately 10 per cent did not allow themselves enough night's rest.[61]

Many people have difficulty starting the day when they are just out of bed. This usually has little to do with problems in objective or subjective sleep duration or quality. It usually is a normal phenomenon called sleep inertia. Our brains have to transition from sleep to wake, and the time to achieve this varies between people. Why did this phenomenon survive evolution? There might be an advantage if it takes a while to wake up properly, because the inertia can help you doze off quickly if you are briefly awake during the night. For most people, feeling sleepy the first half-hour after waking up is normal. Therefore, if you do not feel energised immediately after waking up, it might simply be your brain transitioning from slumber to wake mode.

On edge

It will probably not be a surprise that stress affects your sleep. If you worry a lot, for example, you often do not manage to fall asleep as well. In addition to having negative effects on many aspects of day-time functioning, such as concentration, appetite, mood and sex drive, stress can also have a direct effect on the subjective quality of your sleep and lead to less restful wake. Despite the fact that I now call myself an average sleeper, I still have periods when I am more awake at night and this is often due to stress. A busy day or an important presentation can sometimes cause my sleep to be a little more restless. This will probably be recognisable to many.

There is a clear link between hyperarousal and an increased stress response and chronic insomnia. Stress is a natural response to threats and challenges, and can have a direct negative effect on your night's rest.[62] In a 2008 animal study, neuroscientist Georgina Cano and colleagues placed a number of male rats in separate cages where another male rat had previously been.[63] The smell of the other male was very stressful and the test animals measured less deep sleep and more wakefulness than normal. The study also showed that certain emotion-regulating brain structures remained active, where normally they do not during sleep. In conclusion, when stressed, you sometimes seem to be too active and emotional to have a good night's rest, which shows in the brain.

There is a similar phenomenon in humans. A 2016 study in six countries showed that people who feel less safe in their neighbour-hood experience poorer subjective sleep quality.[64] I myself have been fortunate to always be able to sleep in a relatively safe environment. For me, this has sometimes also led to situations in which it might have been better to wake up sooner. I can remember when my mother woke me up as a child and I half opened my eyes and noticed that my bed was shaking. I heard a lot of noise but apparently, it didn't really alarm me. My mother told me the next day that she woke me up that night because of an earthquake and I just responded with 'Okay' and continued to sleep despite the noise and vibration of the quake. Another example from my adult life was when my bed partner rushed out of bed at night to look out of the bedroom window and tried to wake me up, but couldn't. It turned out that a car was on fire relatively close to my house, causing the neighbours' windows to shatter. I just slept through. Bizarre to think that an earthquake and a blazing fire didn't wake me, but thoughts about not getting enough sleep later often did.

Acute psychosocial stress causes us to take longer to doze off and have reduced subjective sleep quality, especially during the first part of the night.[65] The effects of acute stress on sleep begin to fade after 40–50 minutes, as the physical stress response also begins to dimin-ish. How is it possible that people who experience a lot of stress for a long time often suffer from waking up throughout the night?

The answer probably lies in our thoughts. If we expect more stress (so-called 'anticipatory negative cognitive representations'), we can suffer from this until the later phases of our sleep. For example, if you know that you have to get up very early or are expecting a stress-ful working day, this can lead to reduced sleep quality throughout the night.[66,67] I often saw this in my patients. They'd spend the night worrying about the extent to which their bad night would affect their next day.

In Chapter 1, I stated the important balance between our restorative sleep and having to remain alert at night as a survival mechanism. One study clearly demonstrated how this works physiologically. In 2022, researchers at the University of Salzburg, Austria, examined the brain activity of sleeping subjects while they presented the sound of familiar and unfamiliar voices. The study showed that unfamiliar voices caused alertness responses more often than familiar voices.[68] From this, we can infer that our brain continues to distinguish between familiar and potentially threatening stimuli during the sleep period. This is a good thing. I do not know about you, but I would prefer to react to a strange voice next to me in the bed and not stay asleep.

The ravages of time

Would you like to sleep as well as you did when you were younger? There is a good chance that this wish will not be fulfilled (or not completely fulfilled). This is because your sleep changes as you get older. A reason for this might partly be due to effects of an aging biological clock and a loss of rhythmic functioning. This can lead to more difficulty adjusting to recover from phase shifting, such as in night work.[69] This may lead to more problems initiating and maintaining sleep and in daytime functioning after doing a night shift.

As I mentioned earlier, there is not only a loss in rhythmic functioning, but there is also a shift in the biological clock when you age, which might have an evolutionary explanation. People also become more and more morning-oriented as they get older. Therefore, it is quite normal that your grandmother always got up before the postal worker delivered the morning paper.

Contrary to popular belief, sleep duration remains quite constant from adulthood onwards. More specifically, every 10 years, total sleep time only decreases 8 minutes in males and 10 minutes in females.[70] When reaching 60 years of age, this decrease tends to stabilise.[71] Additional good news is that people above the age of 60 only show minimal changes in the time they need to fall asleep. Furthermore, although arousals occur more frequently in older adults, they maintain their ability to fall asleep as rapidly as young adults.[72,73]

There are distinct alterations in sleep phases while aging. The proportion of NREM1 and NREM2 (both light sleep) increases and the proportion of deep NREM3 and REM dream sleep decreases.[74] In men, there is generally more deterioration of deep sleep than in women.[75]

Although objective measurements might not show shocking differences when aging, subjective sleep shows features that are more distinct in older adults. Up to 50 per cent of older adults report sleep problems.[76] Next to the biological aging of the sleep system, other factors might contribute to this effect as well. For example, poor health and disease burden might create a large proportion of these complaints.[77] Other factors might be being less physically active and receiving less exposure to daylight. In addition, loss of loved ones can lead to emotional distress and loneliness, which can in turn contribute to more subjective sleep problems.[78]

A specific factor that might play a part in worse sleep in aging women is menopause. What causes the specific sleep problems during and after menopause? Poor sleep in this period is not only the result of factors such as aging, night-time hot flashes and changes in psychological functioning. Poor sleep is truly a core symptom of menopause.[79] Problems maintaining sleep are particularly prominent. These problems often persist after menopause and there might be several causes.

The production of the hormones oestrogen and progesterone decreases (further) during this period. Progesterone has an anxiety-reducing and calming effect and has a positive effect on non-REM sleep. A lower progesterone level could therefore logically have a negative effect on sleep. Lower oestrogen appears to go hand in hand with lying awake more often.[80] Oestrogen regulates, among other things, the time of the lowest body temperature at night, and a low oestrogen level is associated with a smaller drop in body temperature.[81] This might lead to a reduction in subjective sleep quality. In addition, nocturnal hot flashes occur in up to 80 per cent of menopausal women. This can lead to waking up drenched in sweat, meaning you have to change your bedding every night. The stronger and more frequent these hot flashes are, the more problems there are in sleeping.[82] Furthermore, mood problems are more common in menopausal women.[83] Sleep may play a role in a vicious circle, with menopausal symptoms disturbing sleep. Waking up more often leads to more night-time worrying, resulting in a gloomy mood or feelings of anxiety. This in turn might have a negative effect on your night's rest.[84] In Chapter 9, I will discuss what might help to combat sleep problems during and after menopause.

Now you know what sleep looks like, how it changes when aging, and how our body manages to keep a good 24-hour rhythm. What happens when a disruption of this process occurs? What are the effects of bad or short sleep? I will address this in the next chapter.

3.

Why Should We Sleep?

'We were given sleep to have a moment's rest from living with
ourselves'[1]

Jacques Deval, *Afin de vivre bel et bien* (1970)

Since antiquity, people have believed that our night's rest has important functions. The ancient Egyptians, as well as the Romans and
Greeks, thought the dreams we experience were gateways through
which they could communicate with the dead and gods. Egyptians
considered nightmares and enigmatic dreams as something supernatural. They built temples to the goddess Isis in which priests gathered
to interpret dreams. Ancient texts and images tell us of dream rituals,[2] whereby a person sleeps in a temple room, and receives healing
or prophetic dreams.

Although we don't have any sources about the role of dreams for
primordial cave dwellers, many contemporary hunter-gatherers do
ascribe a special status to dreams. Some tribes believe that a good
hunter needs to have a strong reciprocal relationship with other species: the animal offers the gift of willing to be approached and
slaughtered, and the human offers rituals, gifts and respect in return.
Some traditional peoples believe that dreaming and trance are ways
of directly communicating with creatures and plants, and that this
enhances the bond with them.[3]

Current theories about sleep have little to do with prophecy and
communication with animals or the dead. Today we focus our

attention not only on the function of dreams but also on the role of sleep as a whole. In particular, sleep appears to play a special role in physical recovery and may be important in reducing energy consumption.[4] Having a good night's rest also appears to have many other benefits, such as leading to better decision-making and supporting our bodily defences.

In this chapter, I'll describe what happens to your body and mind during good sleep and the consequences of bad and short sleep, in particular why when we lie awake at night it can feel like our brain is playing games with us and creating darker thoughts than during the day.

Dead serious

Will you die sooner if you sleep shorter or longer than average? Well, 7 hours of sleep seems to be the golden number and the further away you are from this, the greater the link with mortality. A night's rest of less than 5 hours or more than 9 hours is invariably associated with an increased risk of earlier death.[5,6] As you get older, the relationship between sleep duration and mortality appears to decrease. In people over 65, no connection is found anymore.[7] I often encountered the fear of earlier death in my sleep patients. They had generally read it somewhere that less than 8 hours of sleep would lead to them having shorter life expectancy.

Why do short and long sleepers die earlier? It seems that the mortality link with long duration is stronger.[8,9] An explanation for this might be that long sleepers are more likely to experience other health problems, such as diabetes, cardiovascular disease and obesity.[10] It is not the long sleep itself, but the health problems that could lead to earlier death. Another cause for the link between sleep duration and mortality could be that long, as well as short, sleepers more often have poor sleep quality. Research indeed shows that it is this poor sleep *quality* among short and long sleepers that is associated with a greater risk of earlier death.[11] Therefore, it is important to look not only at the duration but also at the objective and subjective quality of sleep.

So bad sleepers may die earlier. What does that mean for people with insomnia? We know that poor sleep quality is not always the same as insomnia, which can often be a problem of subjective sleep, while objective sleep problems include sleep disorders such as sleep apnoea. It is a comforting idea that the *subjective* sleep problems seen in insomnia alone do not seem to be associated with mortality.[12]

As I mentioned in Chapter 2, studies often poorly define the nature of the measured objective and subjective sleep quality, leading to inaccurate reporting of the relationship between mortality and insomnia. I also described that researchers use measurements from questionnaires that do not distinguish between different sleep problems, such as insomnia and obstructive sleep apnoea.

Unlike insomnia, obstructive sleep apnoea is clearly associated with mortality.[13] Recent research has shown that insomnia is only associated with earlier death when sleep apnoea is also present.[14] An interesting finding here is that often we do not perceive the component of objective sleep quality that is most associated with mortality. This component has to do with a specific kind of sleep fragmentation, namely the short moments in which we wake up and we do not even realise we do (such as in sleep apnoea), and that this is related to dying earlier or later.[15] The general conclusion for people with insomnia is that they do not have to worry about dying earlier due to their sleep problem, and that alone is often a great relief.

What about the impact of varying sleep times and doing shifts? The scientific conclusions are contradictory. Two studies revealed a link between mortality and working evening and night shifts, while other studies show a lack of association between earlier death and working during the night.[16,17,18] It might be that the sex of the individuals, their level of education, and the duration of exposure to evening and night shifts play a role in the relationship with mortality. Male white-collar workers who continue to do night shifts for more than 5 years might have a greater risk of earlier death.[19] Further research is however needed to more clearly establish the relationship between shift work and mortality.

Stay healthy

The assumption that good sleep leads to better health is another idea that dates from antiquity.

In ancient Egypt, people came from far and wide to a temple where they could enter a chamber of dreams – because after a night in such a chamber, their illnesses would surely disappear. In medieval times, physicians believed that a good night's rest showed positive effects on metabolism. They advised lying on your right side during your first sleep to stimulate food digestion. Then in the second sleep, you should sleep on your left side to better calm the body.[20]

Although this sounds a bit like folklore, research shows that the idea of sleeping on a certain side might not be nonsense after all and may have benefits for certain groups of people. For example, if you experience heartburn, such as in gastroesophageal reflux disease (GERD), sleeping on your left side can reduce symptoms.[21] In addition, people with heart failure can experience discomfort from sleeping on their left side, because they can feel the enlarged heart beating against the left chest wall more. Sleeping on the left side might also have a negative effect on the functioning of the heart in this group.[22]

The relationship between sleep and health has become an issue of great concern and debate in modern society. After one short night, you may still feel amazingly well, but if you limit your slumber time too much and for too long, negative physical and psychological effects can occur. What does science say about this?

The difficulty in interpreting the results of studies on sleep duration and health is that research is often based on subjects who have been strongly deprived of sleep in laboratory settings, which translates poorly to real-life situations. In addition, while studies have found a link between sleep duration and certain health problems, researchers have not addressed objective and subjective sleep quality. This is important because, as stated earlier, many people with short sleep also experience problems in sleep quality. The bottom line is that you can only examine the association between sleep and health thoroughly if quality, duration and timing are included in the analysis.[23] In addition, it is important to distinguish between subjective sleep quality problems due to insomnia or objective problems in sleep because of various sleep disorders. Unfortunately, this distinction is often absent in studies on sleep quality and health.

I will now discuss what we *do* know about the relationship between sleep and the most prevalent chronic diseases associated with mortality. Sleep problems are often associated with obesity, which is one of the risk factors for cardiovascular disease. Many people, for instance, think that insomnia can cause you to gain weight or make it harder for you to lose weight. Is there a link between the two?

Researchers have built entire theories around this. For example, people who have their sleep dramatically reduced experience a decrease in leptin (the satiety hormone) and an increase in ghrelin (the hunger hormone). As a result, the need to eat may increase, and there appears to be a preference for eating more carbohydrates and fats.[24] However, researchers often generalise this data to poor sleepers, while studies usually concern good sleepers who experimentally spend only 4 hours in bed. It is incorrect to compare this group to a group of poor sleepers. In fact, a 2017 study showed that there are no differences at all in leptin and ghrelin between people with insomnia and a control group.[25] Myth debunked. Similarly, in 2018, Wai Sze Chan and her colleagues found no clear relationship between insomnia and obesity.[26] On the other hand, there is a link between *extreme* acute sleep deprivation and weight gain, although these effects seem to diminish if the deprivation is continued for a couple of weeks and if the deprivation is milder;[27] the latter is more often the case in real life.

What about the relationship between short sleep, insomnia and another risk factor for cardiovascular problems: hypertension or high blood pressure? Sleep deprivation and going to bed much later than usual might lead to an increased heart rate and high blood pressure. However, the results are contradictory.[28] Patients with insomnia show increased blood pressure and blunting of the normal blood pressure dip.[29] A 2021 meta-analysis by a team of researchers in China showed that early morning awakenings and problems maintaining sleep are associated with increased risk of hypertension, particularly in the European population. The results were not significant for the Asian and American research population; the potential reasons for this difference remain unclear.[30] An important limitation of this research is that several studies did not examine the presence of possible somatic disease, mental health conditions and additional medication use, nor did they look at the individuals' smoking status or socio-economic status. This makes it difficult to conclude whether the risk of developing hypertension is increased by insomnia or by other possible factors.

Diabetes is a disease in which there are defects in insulin secretion, insulin activity or both, which can lead to damage in several organs and pose a risk of developing cardiovascular disease.[31] What is the relationship between diabetes and sleep? Experimental sleep deprivation in average sleepers has shown to reduce insulin sensitivity, which is one of the early indicators of diabetes.[32] Studies on the association between sleep difficulties and prediabetes show contradictory results.[33,34]

In a study looking at objective and subjective measures of sleep difficulties, sleeping less than 5 hours in combination with subjective insomnia complaints was associated with a 300 per cent higher risk of type 2 diabetes. Neither insomnia alone nor short sleep duration alone was associated with the higher risk. Only when the two aspects combined, was there a relationship.[35] What could be a reason for this link? According to a study on insomnia and objective sleep duration, those with short sleep duration were more likely to be older, over-weight, had higher social deprivation scores and more often showed neuropsychiatric disorders. These factors might separately predict the higher incidence of diabetes and explain the relationship between insomnia with objective short sleep and diabetes.[36]

Cardiovascular disease is a widespread public health issue. Risk factors include hypertension, diabetes and obesity. Again, the research shows conflicting results when it comes to the relationship between insomnia and cardiovascular problems.[37] The reason might be that the research population varies a lot between studies. Some studies take factors such as mental health conditions into account, with researchers concluding that depression might be an important factor explaining the link between insomnia and cardiovascular disease. Many people with subjective sleep complaints experience depression, which is an independent risk factor for cardiovascular events.[38]

A 2024 study in almost 3,000 middle-aged women showed that there was a link between insomnia symptoms and cardiovascular disease, irrespective of depressive symptoms.[39] In another study, researchers in the US examined the subjects over a period of 22 years. They concluded that women with chronic severe insomnia symptoms had a 51 per cent higher risk of cardiovascular disease. As I mentioned in Chapter 2, insomnia can be a symptom of sleep apnoea in women. The risk of having sleep apnoea doubles after menopause, which might lead to a high prevalence of the disorder in the examined age group.[40] In addition, the US researchers measured snoring as a possible symptom of sleep apnoea, to estimate whether this disorder might influence the results. However, as also mentioned, snoring is not a good indicator of obstructive sleep apnoea in women and exclusively measuring this symptom leads to underreporting of this disorder, as the researchers confirm in their conclusion.[41] Therefore, the prevalence of this possible underlying disorder and its influence on the results might be underestimated.

In short, because possible clinical diagnoses were not included in the analysis, it is plausible that the risk of cardiovascular events was not elevated by the presence of insomnia, but possibly caused by underlying obstructive sleep apnoea.

Another main cause of death is of course cancer. Can short sleep and insomnia increase the risk of developing certain cancers? Research again shows conflicting results. A 2020 review by Shi showed that insomnia was associated with a 24 per cent higher risk of cancer, and this was only significantly higher for thyroid cancer and for women.[42] According to scientists, the link between insomnia and thyroid cancer might relate to increased thyroid stimulating hormone in this group. However, research on this topic focused on subjects depriving themselves of sleep for 64 hours, which is not comparable to patients suffering from insomnia.[43] Moreover, the 2020 review by Shi warned against early conclusions on possible causality: only a limited number of studies had been made and there was the risk of potential bias.[44] A meta-analysis on a possible association between sleep duration and cancer indicated that neither short nor long sleep duration were associated with increased cancer risk.[45]

All in all, research shows a link between short sleep duration, insomnia and risk factors for cardiovascular ill health such as high blood pressure and diabetes. However, it is not clear whether it is sleeplessness or short sleep causing these problems as there are other factors that might distort a possible association, including: the presence of a possible depressive disorder or other mental health conditions; the use of sleep medication; the presence of possible (other) somatic disease.

For cancer, there was no association found with short or long sleep duration; it is difficult to draw firm conclusions on a possible causal relationship between insomnia and the disease. In short, the hypothesised causal links between insomnia, short sleep and chronic disease are not as straightforward as previously suggested.

Although there are many more health problems than I have described above, these findings might be quite reassuring for biologically based short sleepers and patients suffering from insomnia.

Immunity

Are you more likely to get sick if you do not sleep well? And the other way around: can you sleep yourself back to health? It would seem so. In fact, your night's rest plays an important role in your bodily defences. The immune system is a network in the body which defends against illnesses. It is important that the system is strong enough to defend when necessary but also that it is not constantly in defence mode, because this can create autoimmune responses such as allergies, which can also have negative health consequences.

Your body enters a kind of reserve state when you sleep, leaving energy for all kinds of important bodily processes. During deep sleep, for example, the release of so-called cytokines peaks. These substances are important because they help you fight off nasty viruses and bacteria. So, if you have been sitting next to someone with a bad cold today, you had better get a good night's rest to prevent a possible viral infection.

Another way in which your sleep affects your immune system is through the proliferation of immune cells.[46] Those cells can be thought of as internal guard dogs that bite every bacterium and virus in the calves. Therefore, it makes sense that poor sleepers are more vulnerable to viruses or infections.[47]

In addition, the deeper you sleep, the better your immune response. This conclusion follows from research on the effectiveness of hepatitis A vaccinations. The subjects' immune systems responded better after a night's sleep than after being awake overnight after the vaccination. In particular, deep sleep was associated with a good immune response.[48]

The immune system can also be too active, which might lead to allergies. Scientists found that a disruption of your biological clock, such as going to bed too late, might increase the likelihood of an allergic response.[49] This disturbance could lead to altered hormone levels and induce hypersensitivity of the skin. Research in mice showed that a different 24-hour rhythmicity of levels of the hormone corticosterone because of biological clock problems might induce skin allergies.[50] Therefore, when you are suffering from allergies, consistently timing your sleep to match your biological clock might help reduce the symptoms. Lack of sleep can also have an effect on the expression of allergic reactions. For example, individuals with peanut allergies were found to be more susceptible to an allergy attack after sleep deprivation.[51]

In summary, there is evidence that a good sleep can support your immune system and that it is important for maintaining an immune response that is both strong enough when needed but not too reactive in everyday situations.

Gaining muscle

You may have noticed that you perform less well at the gym or while running if you've slept poorly. This is not surprising, because sleep and physical performance are closely related. Sleep plays an important role in the maintenance of muscle tissue. From population data, we know that there is an association between chronic insufficient sleep, or subjective poor-quality sleep, and lower muscle mass.[52] Whether the poor sleep quality was related to subjective sleep difficulties due to insomnia or symptoms possibly due to obstructive sleep apnoea was not specified. Furthermore, a night of complete sleep deprivation or a disrupted biological clock can lead to an increase of muscle breakdown.[53,54] Research suggests that the negative effects of 5 nights of sleep deprivation is just as large as the decrease in muscle protein synthesis after a short-term energy restriction.[55,56] Thus, sleeping less can have a similar effect on our muscles as eating less. It is important to note that the deprivation of sleep was strong in these experiments, with a maximum sleep opportunity of 4 hours for the research participants. This is not comparable to the smaller sleep deprivation many people put themselves through in real life.

What is the mechanism behind this? How can the lack of sleep have a negative effect on our muscle tissue? A dysregulation of anabolic hormones might contribute to this. Anabolic hormones include testosterone, GH and IGF-1; they regulate muscle tissue growth and repair.[57] For example, after one night of sleep deprivation researchers found that there was a 24 per cent decrease of testosterone levels in healthy males and females.[58] In contrast, after better sleep there is an increase in the anabolic hormone IGF-1.[59] Good subjective sleep quality is also associated with greater muscle strength.[60] Sleep duration seems to matter more in young men than in young women. A study of college students showed that only shorter-sleeping men (less than 6 hours of sleep) have lower muscle strength than average- to longer-sleeping men (more than 7 hours of sleep), while in women there was no difference.[61] In middle-aged and older adults, sleep duration might also impact muscle strength, but research results are inconclusive.[62] Another study found that, as you age, sleep quality rather than sleep duration becomes especially important for maintaining muscle strength and muscle mass.[63] Here a broad measure of sleep quality was used, which makes it difficult to interpret the results and whether possible insomnia symptoms or symptoms associated with sleep disorders such as obstructive sleep apnoea might have the greatest effect on the results.

Painkiller

There is a clear relationship between pain experience and sleep. Researchers estimate that many people with chronic pain suffer from broken nights on a regular basis: 24–34 per cent suffer from chronic insomnia, which is almost double the prevalence in the general population.[64]

You may think that sleep complaints are always the result of pain complaints and not the other way around. It is logical that the experience of back pain or a headache might keep you awake. However, the relationship appears to be more complex. In fact, poor sleep predicts chronic pain complaints rather than vice versa. More specifically, in a large 2013 review, researchers at the Johns Hopkins University School of Medicine in Baltimore found that insomnia symptoms increase the likelihood of future chronic headache or migraine, while these problems did not necessarily predict the onset of insomnia.[65] People who, in addition to chronic pain, also suffer from insomnia experience more severe pain, longer-lasting pain complaints and experience a greater negative effect on daily functioning.[66]

It seems that disturbed sleep has a negative effect on the experience of pain. Further, treatment of sleep disorders might help alleviate pain-related symptoms. If people with pain complaints also receive sleep therapy in addition to pain treatment, there is less daily disruption due to pain and patients indicate that they are less tired and depressed.[67] So if you suffer from pain complaints, make sure that you are not only treated for the pain, but that attention is also paid to your subjective sleep quality.

What is the background to these findings? An explanation for this relationship is that poor sleep increases sensitivity to painful stimuli. For example, one study showed that more sleep problems due to pain led to more sensitivity to electrical pain stimuli.[68] At the same time, stress and concerns about your health can worsen insomnia symptoms. The hypothesis is that these worries create excessive alertness, which leads to less subjective quality sleep.[69] A body in pain ends up in the evolutionary survival mode and that leads to you checking the environment for danger sooner. This alert mode does not help to achieve a good night's rest.

Do not forget to sleep

Do you ever suffer from forgetfulness after a bad night? You may have noticed that acquiring new information does not go so well if you had a bad sleep the night before. Sleep problems are often associated with concentration problems and with difficulties in learning. That is something I recognise. If I sleep worse at night, all kinds of things go wrong. I even had the experience of rushing to work after a rough night, then at lunch after a long morning, it was pointed out that I had a sock hanging down the back of my trousers. I'd overslept and quickly put on my trousers in haste while forgetting that my sock from the day before was still in them. The psychological assistant who drew my attention to the sock reminded me of this incident for months to come.

Your memory contains different parts. For example, when you memorise a number of words, you use a different part of the brain to when you learn to ride a bicycle. Declarative memory concerns learning factual knowledge while non-declarative memory concerns learning skills. German psychologist Hermann Ebbinghaus, who in a study tried to memorise nonsense words, described the connection between declarative memory and sleep as early as 1885. He found that recalling this information was better if he had slept well beforehand.[70]

Sleep affects the functioning of both declarative and non-declarative memory. For declarative memory, NREM3 sleep seems to play a particularly important role. In your deep sleep, you probably reactivate a previously learned connection so that the information is better stored in our brain.[71] That is why it is not wise for students to try to study until late the night before an exam: they barely get a good night's sleep or do not sleep at all; they then take their seats in the exam room to begin their test with red-flushed eyes. It is wise to get enough restful sleep after studying. Are you currently studying? Then make sure you stop learning in the evening on time and go do something that relaxes you. Do not go to bed too early, else your sleep pressure will not be high enough. Also, try not to go to bed too late, so that you have enough sleep to 'rock' your exam. If you have a presentation at work the next day, it is also better not to practise it too late in the evening and to use the end of the day for relaxation.

In non-declarative memory, both deep sleep and REM sleep play important roles. The improvement of your skills is probably 'recorded' in our brain during deep sleep. REM sleep then acts as a kind of 'amplifier' of this memory.[72] Therefore, if you are taking a course in macramé or advanced hula-hooping, sleep will help you apply the skill you have just learned even better in the future.

By the way, when it comes to learning new things, not only night-time sleep might contribute. A 30-minute nap during the day can have as much positive effect on your ability to learn as a full night's sleep.[73] However, try to limit the time of napping, and don't nap in the evening, because this can have negative effects on your sleep pressure and thus your sleep. Most experts recommend napping no later than 8 hours before going to bed. It is also important not to lie in bed, but to choose, say, an easy chair or sofa. It is best to associate the bed with night sleep as much as possible.

A specific term that comes into mind when talking about memory and memory problems is dementia. It is a general term for the impaired ability to think, or make decisions, which interferes with daily life. Usually, one of the most prominent features is loss of memory functions. There are different kinds of dementia. One of the most prevalent is Alzheimer's disease, the early stages of which affect 22 per cent of all people aged 50 and above worldwide.[74]

A recent large review showed an association between sleep problems and an increased risk of developing Alzheimer's. Overall, the risk of developing cognitive impairment or Alzheimer's is 1.68 times higher for people with sleep problems than those without. However, 'sleep problems' is again a very broad definition of all kinds of symptoms and disorders. More explicitly, the nature of the studied sleep problems varied strongly between the reviewed studies. Some studies measured sleep quality by looking at obstructive sleep apnoea and others by using a questionnaire that measured insomnia complaints as well as sleep apnoea. The link between obstructive sleep apnoea and Alzheimer's disease is clear, because disruptions in sleep due to loss of oxygen and comorbid cardiovascular problems pose a clear risk of developing the disease.[75] Therefore, a lack of distinction between different sleep problems might give people the (wrong) impression that insomnia is one of the important causes of Alzheimer's.

Although research shows a possible link between insomnia and the onset of Alzheimer's, it often does not review various factors which might have an influence on this tentative relationship.[76] One of these factors is the use of sleep medication, the most common of which are benzodiazepines. Evidence suggests that exposure to or use of benzodiazepines might increase the risk of developing Alzheimer's and that the link between insomnia and Alzheimer's is distorted by the negative influence of this type of sleep medication.[77,78] Indeed, in 2012 Taiwanese researchers showed that there is a relationship between using (more) sleep medication (benzodiazepines and nonbenzodiazepines, such as Zopiclone and Zolpidem) and an increased risk of Alzheimer's disease.[79] However, specifically benzodiazepine use does not seem to explain the link between insomnia and Alzheimer's completely.[80]

Another important factor that poses a problem in defining a causal relationship is that sleep problems are often an early sign of Alzheimer's and that it might not be that insomnia causes it, but that sleeplessness is merely a symptom of a very early stage of the disease.[81] In summary, it is not clear whether insomnia is one of the causes of Alzheimer's, while the relationship between obstructive sleep apnoea and Alzheimer's is much clearer.

Another interesting link between dementia and our night's rest concerns interventions that might help combat Alzheimer's disease. Interventions during sleep might play a role in decreasing the progression of the disease. Research shows that exposing patients with Alzheimer's to scents of aromatic oils during their sleep might help counter the disease process. That may sound a bit crazy, but on second thought, it is not. The olfactory system is the only sensory system in the brain with direct projections to the limbic system, which is very important for memory and emotion.[82]

In dementia, one of the first symptoms is often the decline of the sense of smell, even before memory problems occur. In fact, loss of smell can predict loss of grey matter in the hippocampus, a structure that is very important for our memory. Research shows that olfactory stimulation counters cognitive decline and people with dementia had strong improvements in memory, attention and language skills, among other things, after exposure to different scents.[83,84] That effect occurred after fifteen days. Exposing patients with dementia to scents during sleep led to better memory performance for 6 months. One study also indicates that a brain structure that probably plays a role in episodic memory and language showed positive changes after the exposure.[85] This brain structure, the uncinate fasciculus, deteriorates in aging and furthermore in Alzheimer's cases. It seems that the exposure to scents might counteract this degeneration.

Obviously, prehistoric man did not know of a relationship between Alzheimer's and olfactory stimulation, but the question is whether it would have been of much use. Primordial man did not live that long and the chance that he was confronted with age-related diseases such as Alzheimer's is very small. For us increasingly older people, it would be interesting to investigate on an even larger scale whether administering scents during sleep can play an important role in combating cognitive decline in people with dementia.

Dream on

In ancient times, people thought that dreams would help them make good choices. According to tradition, this was already the case with Alexander the Great, who reigned between 336–323 BCE. When he was besieging the city of Tyros (modern-day Tyre, in Lebanon), he dreamed of a satyr, a mythical forest creature, dancing on a shield. A dream interpreter recognised a play on words in the dream, namely '*Sa Tyros*', meaning 'Tyros is yours'. Not long after having the dream, Alexander conquered the ancient city.[86]

Historically, there were a number of inventors and scientists who may have experienced a 'eureka moment' just after waking up. For example, it is said that the Russian chemist Dmitri Mendeleev first described the periodic table of elements one morning after an insightful dream, although some say the story is apocryphal.[87] (I never dream about chemistry, and somehow I am glad. I like a little night flying above the clouds a lot better.) Even the term eureka has its own origin story. Archimedes is said to have shouted it when he got into the bath and discovered that the water was rising. According to the Roman architect Vitruvius, Archimedes concluded that the amount of water risen must be equal to the volume of his body. Pretty clever! (When I take a bath, I just put on some nice music, and I'm not so concerned with the rising water level.) On a side note, Vitruvius described this event about 200 years after it was supposed to have happened, so he may have been wrong. Stories change over time, especially if they were not written down and are passed down from generation to generation.[88]

Back to dreaming! A nice dream can be an amazing experience: you lie down looking at all the beautiful colourful images. Then the alarm clock goes off. You can reminisce about what you just dreamed, but after a few seconds, you forget your dream! If our sleep is so important for our memory, why do we forget our dreams?

The reason for this is that you have lower levels of norepinephrine in your brain during and just after REM (dream) sleep.[89] This substance is important for our memory. This is why you can only remember your dream when directly waking up from REM sleep and thereafter forget the dream quickly. What is the function of forgetting your dreams? For the survival of our species, remembering dreams was probably of little use. Dreams are mostly compilations of previous impressions. Our brain creates combined sensations during your dream of things you've seen, heard or felt. You use your memory in the process. This is also why you cannot dream in clear intense images if you are born blind. You have never seen anything, so your brain has not been able to store visual information and there is no input for any dream images. Therefore, dreams are mostly old memories in a new guise. They can express themselves in a beautiful form or a terrible one. You can dream about deceased people with whom you had a good bond or about unpleasant moments such as that exam you failed. Dreams can go in any direction.

While deep sleep seems to be especially important for physical recovery and basic memory functions, REM sleep is important for processing emotions and emotional memory. A well-functioning body that recovers is important for immediate survival, but scientists discovered that our REM sleep has an important function in higher cognitive skills, creativity and solution-oriented ability, especially in creating new associations.[90] In line with this, creativity and problem-solving abilities increase after a good night's rest. Sleep leads you to see connections more easily and quickly.[91] A complex problem you might face before you go to bed suddenly seems to disappear like snow before the sun. As Meat Loaf sang in his song 'Paradise by the Dashboard Light', sleeping on something can contribute to better choices, possibly even when it comes to choosing a partner.

If you create the right sleep conditions, you can even force a eureka moment. In fact, if you smell a certain scent during the day while trying to solve a problem, it helps to diffuse that same scent in your bedroom. Perceiving that smell while you sleep leads to more creativity and choosing better solutions when you are awake.[92] The association between the scent and the problem you want to solve is apparently enough to prompt your brain to start working on it at night. That way you have already done some 'preliminary work' without much effort. Therefore, if you are remodelling a house and you are not sure if you should demolish a load-bearing wall, you can place a nice lavender scent among the debris. You put that same lavender scent next to your bed at night. At least then in the morning you will know for sure if the construction of your house will hold up. (You might also want to check the original construction blueprint just to be sure . . .)

As humans, we do not have claws or a great running speed, so we mainly rely on our cognitive skills. In fact, you can only get excited when you consider that dreams are an opportunity to go off the beaten track. You can enter into limitless new situations in a virtual reality world that your brain creates itself.

One hypothesis is that during dreams our brain mainly tries to create situations accompanied by high emotions. In fact, the amygdala, a brain structure that particularly gives emotional value to situations, becomes very active during REM sleep.[93] This is why dreams are often very emotional. Sometimes people can even wake up crying because the experience has been so intense. It can also feel frustrating or irritating after waking up from a dream.

The threat hypothesis, which I will discuss further in Chapter 10, assumes that we can practise endlessly with situations that are important or threatening to us. At the same time, there is evidence that the eye movements we make could contribute to the extinction of emotional responses. Indeed, one study indicated that eye movements can down-regulate the amygdala.[94] Therefore, hypothetically, our brain turns on the emotion machine and the emotion-processing machine at the same time. Why? Probably because it makes us smarter when confronted with threatening situations. If we reduce the high negative emotional value of a more complex or chronic threatening situation, we can plan better. An overly emotional brain does not think very well!

In short: your dreams are useful and perhaps dreaming has even been more important for survival of the human species than you might think! Primordial man may have benefited from deep sleep for immediate survival, but the REM dream sleep probably led him to come up with long-term solutions for impending danger, such as ways of taking shelter or planning certain routes for journeys from one place to another.

Evidence for this theory comes from research on the dream content of the Hadza in Tanzania and the BaYaka, hunter-gatherers in the Congo Basin. In 2023, Professor Samson and colleagues compared their dreams to the dreams of people living in industrialised societies.[95] They found the BaYaka dreamed more about others in their community when they were experiencing interpersonal conflict in their day-to-day lives. At that time, the BaYaka revealed they were in conflict with neighbouring Bantu fisher-farmers over trading. Research suggests that for the BaYaka, community-orientated dreams – about family and friends, receiving social support – is helpful because these people rely more on others to cope with their specific daily threats. One of the tribe members had a dream about net hunting with her family and catching many animals, or working together with the others. For the Hadza, daily threats are less caused by neighbouring communities than by predators and wild animals. An example of a Hadza dream was a tribe member describing how he was chased by a herd of elephants and had to hide in a cave.

In general, external threat content in dreams was higher in both the Hadza and BaYaka when compared to the individuals examined in industrialised societies in Switzerland, Belgium and Canada. In a subgroup of students during the COVID-19 pandemic, the content of the dreams was more about confronting daily challenges alone and social isolation, which may reflect the specific fears the students faced during that period. The scientists concluded that dreams can effectively regulate emotions by linking potential threats with non-fearful contexts.[96] These dreams might help reduce anxiety and negative emotions, leading to better and more thoughtful solutions.

Vivid dreams are not always pleasant. An example: you are walking down a narrow dark corridor. You do not know where you are. You hear a noise behind you and realise that something is wrong. You start walking faster and you feel rushed. Cautiously you look back and see a shadow that grows larger and larger. Panic strikes. You feel your heart pounding and you want to get away, but you cannot escape. Bathed in sweat, you wake up. It was a nightmare. Moments later, you can recall exactly what you dreamed.

Why is it that you can often remember nightmares? It probably has to do with how your memory works. You remember emotionally charged information better. Evolutionarily, neutral or positive dreams may not have been that important, but emotionally charged dreams were probably relevant to our survival. Evolutionarily, neutral or positive dreams do not help you cope better with danger or threat and therefore you are unlikely to remember them. If you remembered all your dreams, it would put an unnecessary burden on your memory. Forgetting them leaves room to store more important information. Nightmares helped us deal with danger. Exactly how that works, I'll explain in Chapter 10.

By the way, there is a way to remember dreams better. Keep a notebook next to your bed and write any down as you wake up. This practice is centuries old. We know from surviving papyrus documents that ancient Egyptians wrote down their dreams.[97] For example, there is a famous dream book from 1275 BCE, which you can see with your own eyes at the British Museum in London. There are still many people who value writing down and explaining dreams.

From the perspective of sleep science, I just wonder whether we are meant to remember most dreams. If remembering dreams were important for survival, it does not make sense that we forget most of them quite quickly after waking. Later in this book I will give some examples where it can be useful to write down certain dreams.

Out of bed on the wrong foot

Over a hundred years ago, Sigmund Freud was concerned with the relationship between our psychological functioning and sleep. He analysed dreams just as the dream interpreters of classical antiquity did, but there was an important difference. Namely, Freud did not believe that dreams were a means of communication between the living and the dead, but that they originated from our subconscious.[98] Dreams, he asserted, were expressions of distorted and unconscious desires. Freud engaged in dream interpretation to make those desires clear and conscious. According to him, emotions such as repressed anger or fear became visible in this way, leading to healing of all kinds of psychological complaints. Today, explaining dreams receives less attention in the world of psychotherapy, but there are regular studies on the link between sleep and emotions. Poor sleep can lead to irritability and mood swings. Therefore, the next time you throw a tantrum during a meeting because the coffee is lukewarm, you could always use a poor night's rest as an excuse. In any case, I think it's good if people are occasionally more open about how they function after a bad night. It can sometimes help in communication if others around you know how you feel at work or at home. On the other hand, I think it's about balance. As a sleep therapist, I sometimes saw patients who talked a lot about their bad sleep. When you talk about it a lot, you give it a lot of attention and in some cases this can also make the problem worse.

To understand how sleep affects your emotions, it is important to know that an emotion consists of two dimensions: value and arousal. The value has to do with how positive or negative the emotion is. The arousal says something about the intensity of the emotion; it can be low, medium or high. Imagine you are standing bewildered in front of the mirror because you are having a 'bad hair day'. The value of your emotion at that moment is probably slightly negative and your arousal medium. Now if you have that exciting date tonight and your hair is a complete mess, the intensity of your emotion may just quickly increase, with accompanying heightened arousal. I do have an example from my own life when I'm in traffic. If I have someone in front of me who drives much slower than the permitted speed, it can sometimes irritate me. The value of my emotion is negative and the arousal is quite low. If I then have to slam on the brakes because the same person is not properly assessing a traffic situation, my arousal can increase considerably. Of course I could also put a nice song on the radio and increase my following distance, but that solution does not always come to mind at such a moment.

In particular the memory for the emotional value of what you sense is enhanced through good sleep.[99] Suppose you come across a place or an object that triggers a negative emotion. Perhaps rummaging through your nightstand you find a picture of your ex? When you go to sleep, chances are that the next time you see that picture; you will feel those same emotions just as intensely. However, if you see that photo again later that same day you will react to it a lot less violently. Sleep preserves the connection between information and the emotional value of that information. Although, of course, the key question really is, why do you still have a picture of your ex in your nightstand?

Subjective sleep quality can also affect your mood. In a scientific study, neutral images, such as neutral faces and household items, were rated more negatively after a sleepless night.[100] So the next time you walk past your vacuum cleaner and feel an irresistible urge to kick it, you may be suffering the consequences of another unpleasant night. Sleep deprivation can cause you to place more emphasis on the negative things that happen to you over the positive things. You judge what you perceive or experience more negatively. It also has other negative effects. Most of us are good at analysing facial expressions. You often know exactly whether your partner, your kids, the dog, the baker, the bank teller or your boss are looking happy or disapproving. This helps you assess social situations. Sleep deprivation makes you more likely to perceive facial expressions as threatening.[101] So if that always-friendly cashier whom you stand before twice a week at the cash register suddenly turns into a grumpy person, you know what's going on. You must have had a bad night.

Maybe you recognise the situation in which you cannot doze off and, after a while, you start ruminating and thinking more negatively about situations you encountered the day or weeks before. What is the reason for this? You might be dealing with a phenomenon called *mind after midnight*. The mind after midnight hypothesis states that psychological complaints appear to increase after 12 a.m.[102] People are more likely to think negatively, worry, and make impulsive and poor decisions when their biological clock indicates they should be sleeping. For most people, the absolute low point is between 2 a.m. and 3 a.m. Studies indicate that suicides are more likely to occur around this time, with the risk of someone taking their own life three times higher at night.[103] Researchers think that more impulsive decision-making plays a role in this extremely elevated risk. It seems that people with suicidal thoughts can become overwhelmed by negative emotions and feel even less control over their own life circumstances at night.

It is important to note that the absolute low point may be a little later for evening people and earlier for morning people. The 'mind after midnight' hypothesis describes how our emotional processing, decision making and impulse control are most disturbed at that moment.

How does that work in our brain? According to the 'synaptic homeostasis hypothesis', staying awake for too long leads to disrupted transmission of signals in our brain. This reduces the effectiveness of cortical functioning (that part of the brain with which we think and organise, among other things). There is also an increase in dopaminergic activation, which can trigger symptoms of impulse control, sensation-seeking and a disturbed sense of reality.[104]

Being awake during the night might sound awful, but the other, more positive side of the story is that many people indicate that they are most creative at night. That would also fit the hypothesis, because less inhibition of thought would lead to a creative mind that is more likely to think outside the box. There is less cognitive control, so more room for creativity. Think of the artists and people with other occupations who work late into the night. Being awake at night can lead to a more positive or negative turn in your mind, depending on a number of factors (including, for example, your predisposition for negative feelings).

The conclusion is that our brain seems to work differently during the night and there appears to be less control over behaviour, thoughts and emotions. However, researchers should further test this hypothesis through empirical studies. Anyhow, the old saying, 'It is best to sleep on it', seems to contain some truth.

Insomnia elevates the risk of developing mental health conditions. Among other things, it is associated with a higher risk of depression, anxiety and alcohol abuse.[105] This link is bidirectional, which means it goes both ways. Mental health conditions can often cause sleep problems as well. For example, traumatic events and post-traumatic stress disorder (PTSD) can have an effect on the night's rest. As a sleep therapist I often worked with people with past traumas and saw this reflected: people who, logically, did not seem to feel safe enough to surrender to sleep after traumatising events. Not only are nightmares a symptom of PTSD, but fear of sleep can also play a role in a hyperactive body that wants to remain able to respond to possible threats.[106] If you look at this from the perspective of prehistoric man and his living conditions, it is understandable. If you grow up in a very unsafe situation, your body will adapt to the unsafe situation and the body may therefore pay more attention to immediate survival.

While somewhere in evolution short-term insomnia could have been adaptive to deal with this threat, the chronic insomnia in many people with PTSD seems to be a consequence of the state of high arousal of the body that is deeply stored. This is also called the lack of 'fear extinction'.[107] In Chapter 9, I will mention a powerful method that might help counteract insomnia in the case of comorbid mental health conditions. I think it is important to try these evidence-based techniques because research shows they often help. However, my experience with thousands of patients is that this sometimes does not help in people who suffer from the effects of early or complex trauma. In this case, it is good to go back to the drawing board and investigate why it does not work. Sometimes a health professional can help in making this analysis and traumatised people might learn to experience a feeling of safety in body and mind again.

As I stated earlier, depression and insomnia often occur together. About 75 per cent of people with depression sleep poorly and 1 in 8 chronically poor sleepers experience depression.[108] Untreated insomnia is associated with a four times higher risk of a depressive disorder.[109] Where does that correlation come from?

In 2012, Dieter Rieman and colleagues described how activation of the arousal system in our brain is an important characteristic of both depression and insomnia; but there is more.[110] Even the sleep structure is different among poor sleepers, which expresses itself in a longer but also more fragmented REM sleep.[111,112]

What is special is that almost all antidepressants suppress REM sleep. In fact, the more these agents do this, the stronger the positive therapeutic effect.[113] What could be the reason for this? REM sleep plays an important role in emotional memory, and a theory is that this phase strengthens negative memories and their interpretation. This can cause you to end up in a negative 'loop'.

According to a review about brain mechanisms in insomnia by the Dutch researcher E. J. van Someren, fragmented REM sleep impedes overnight emotional regulation and those with fragmented REM sleep became more sensitive to stress. He concludes that these patients might have even been better off without REM sleep. Indeed, the fragmentation of REM sleep as seen in patients with depression and insomnia might even be a predisposing factor for the development of both disorders.[114,115]

Reducing REM sleep could therefore lead to more room for perspective and alternative interpretations of emotional memories and that could lead to a better mood. In this way, it might make people less susceptible to developing (more) depressive symptoms. Because many people with depressive complaints are more inactive and often stay in bed longer, this can lead to relatively more (fragmented) REM sleep. This can further perpetuate the negative loop. In fact, shortening total bed times can be a powerful way to reduce symptoms of depression. A meta-analysis of 8 studies showed that shorter total bed time and more sleep deprivation can lead to mood elevation in people with depression. However, this improvement is often short-lived, with a positive effect seen in the first 2 weeks only.[116]

Not only the structure but also the timing of sleep appears to be important in the development of depressive symptoms. At almost every level in our body, including the cell, neuronal and organ levels, there are time-sensitive mechanisms that keep a balance. A theory is that these mechanisms are out of step in depression. Working shifts or having jet lag are among some of the factors thought to trigger this. For example, it appears that nurses who work night shifts are at increased risk of experiencing depression.[117]

To sum up, it seems that there is a strong link between mood and sleep, and that insomnia or sleep deprivation can lead to long-term problems with psychological functioning. Therefore, it is very important to look at the subjective quality of sleep and to reducing restless wakefulness when people are facing psychological stress or showing symptoms of a mental health condition. Improving the night's rest might enhance psychological recovery mechanisms and lead to better daytime functioning.

In this chapter, I discussed the effects of sleep on health and daily functioning – but what happens exactly when you experience sleep-lessness and what can you do to restore your night's rest? In the next chapters, I will focus on the effects of insomnia on daily functioning and the essentials for improving our night's rest.

4.

Sleepless Nights

'Sleep is the only friend who does not come when called'[1]

Comtesse Diane de Beausacq, *Maximes de la vie* (1883)

A relevant question now is: did primordial peoples suffer from insomnia? If their attitude towards sleepless nights was the same as that of the contemporary hunter-gatherers, then most likely not! Among today's traditional peoples, the idea of 'insomnia' does not appear to be in their vocabulary. In fact, only 1.5 to 2.5 per cent of tribal members indicate that they regularly have trouble dozing off or maintaining sleep.[2] As I discussed in Chapter 2, although they lie awake much longer than we do, the Hadza don't see waking up in between sleep, or falling asleep late, as a problem. This is of course a very different attitude to what we in industrialised societies have been brought up with, and it can be a relief for people who struggle with their sleep every night.

A more neutral approach to night-waking was probably also true for primordial humans, and perhaps they even saw the positive aspects of a broken night. Wild animals or hostile tribes could rob them of their sleep, but in that case, more fragmented nights served a clear purpose: survival. In prehistoric times, individual sleep differences must have been beneficial for survival of the group. As discussed in Chapter 1, differences in natural circadian rhythms might have helped us. The evening types were alert until late, and the morning types could be alert early in the morning.

However, that could not have covered the whole night. A theory is that light sleepers filled the gaps in between, being able to react relatively quickly to danger even as they slumbered. As a result, someone could always alert the others to danger. It may be a cold comfort to the people with insomnia, but they were probably the superheroes of the cave dwellers.

That is personal

Almost everyone has a bad night from time to time. Stress about a deadline, financial problems, relationships, an exam or important appointment can cause you to stare at the ceiling all night. Usually, this only affects a few nights. If it lingers on, you may just find yourself suffering from chronic insomnia.

Insomnia is very common. Twenty per cent of the population experiences occasional insomnia and about 10 per cent of the population has chronic insomnia.[3] It occurs nearly 1½ times more in women than in men; I will elaborate more on this gender difference later in this chapter.[4] Chronic insomnia includes problems initiating or maintaining sleep at least three nights a week and/or waking up too early. A combination of these problems often occurs. However, the effects (and conditions) of insomnia are not limited to the night.

To meet the criteria for a diagnosis of insomnia, daytime symptoms must also be present. Examples are concentration and memory problems, fatigue and reduced daytime functioning.[5] People suffering from insomnia are often less productive at home and at work, and sometimes no longer feel like meeting up socially with others.

I have experienced these problems first hand. My own fragmented nights became a struggle. I had been sleeping poorly for 2 or 3 years and could not figure out what was causing these problems. Before, I really looked forward to my bed, but I started to dread the nights more and more. During those dark hours, my thoughts were racing. I would look at my phone and watch the hours of the night slowly pass. I regularly got out of bed and then felt miserable, tired and sometimes nauseous. I could no longer relax. I was working on a theatre performance during that year, teaching a group of twenty dancers a choreography for Georges Bizet's opera *Carmen*. The music and dance steps of a choreography were stuck in my head. I did not understand what was going on. I had a nice life, good health, loving relationship, nice work and good contact with my colleagues. My life was running smoothly and still I could not sleep.

Being a sleep therapist who could not manage to create a good night's rest for himself embarrassed me. It was a big step to visit my doctor, but I decided to make an appointment anyway. The GP nodded understandingly and referred me to a psychotherapist. The therapist advised me to watch television prior to sleeping because he had read in an article that it might take my mind of things and create more mental peace. That was surprising advice, because I kept telling my clients that the best thing to do was to get the TV out of the bedroom. On the other hand, it was not that surprising at all, because like many people with insomnia, I was not able to fall asleep in bed, but while watching television in the evening I sometimes dozed off. My therapist told me that I was probably asking too much of myself. The advice around watching TV helped me a bit. After going to bed, I turned it on and noticed that I'd fall asleep faster. When I motivated myself to apply shorter total bed times through 'sleep restriction' (which I will discuss in Chapter 9) my problems decreased further and I experienced even more restful nights.

After a couple of years, when the theatre show was over, my sleep problems vanished completely. I regained peace of mind. Apparently, the preparations for that performance had made me too active to rest well during the night. I also saw this mental hyperactivity a lot in my patients. I treated people who were too busy during the day and then expected to sleep like a baby at night. The only big difference was that I was mainly positively active, while my patients were often plagued by negative mental hyperactivity. The exact mechanism behind this remained a mystery until I delved into evolutionary psychology. That helped me answer the 'why' question. Why had I slept so badly for so long?

I understood my clients better because of my own experiences with insomnia. Headlines like 'Short sleep leads to earlier death', and 'Why you need 8 hours of sleep', but also quick conclusions from research articles and books on this matter, bothered me. A flashy headline sometimes seemed more important than a critical scientific view. Moreover, I noted that the fear of not being able to sleep well only increases when you read such reports. These headlines are not only bad for your sleep; they often depict a distorted reality or are not evidence-based.

Besides the frightening reports from the media, you also have to deal with well-meant advice from those around you, which can drive you to despair. 'Maybe you should just not worry so much', 'You should just let it go', and 'Ah, I sleep badly sometimes, too.' Such comments often backfire. You feel powerless when, in your opinion, you have tried everything and your sleep problem still does not diminish. It is also difficult when other people don't seem to realise how tough it can be to have a sleep problem. Some people are lighthearted or giggly about it. If you are a good sleeper yourself, it is of course difficult to imagine how poor sleep can affect your life. If you have busy days in which you want to be alert and perform well, this is often difficult to achieve after bad nights.

When you experience insomnia, you often dread the night. The bedroom becomes a place that reminds you of all those nights before. Every time you lie down in bed, that one thought comes to you: 'Will *it* work tonight?' As a result, you may be tempted to avoid the bed and just doze off on the couch. Alternatively, you go to bed much earlier because you think this might help you get more sleep.

My clients tried all sorts of things in the fight against their insomnia. They bought overpriced mattresses and bedding; they drank warm milk with honey; they tried meditation. Many had been to various counsellors who tried to create a better night's sleep through acupuncture, herbs, potions and dowsing rods. Often it was all in vain.

People with insomnia often have a partner who sleeps very well. There is nothing more annoying than the sound of your husband or wife snoring while you are counting sheep. Counting sheep is of course something most people with insomnia don't do. Usually, they are more concerned about anything and everything else, and especially about their own sleep.

Those partners, by the way, often felt almost as helpless as the patient did. 'How did you sleep?', they would ask in the morning, to which they would usually get the irritated response: 'I slept terribly, and you?'

The vicious circle

As we've seen, through evolution the structure of our sleep has probably adapted to the possibility of external threats in the night. Most deep NREM3 sleep occurs in the first half of the night, which means that after half of your sleep time, you've already had the most important sleep for direct survival. This means that our bodies can recover through sleep in a relatively short period, which leads to lengthening of the wake period in which we can react to external threats. Another characteristic that could help us survive is that you have a period of light sleep in between the deeper stages. This makes it easier to wake up between deep phases and scan your surroundings for possible danger. If you spend hours just sleeping deeply, you are an easy target for sabre-toothed tigers and bears.

Nowadays it is especially useful to wake up if you have to go to the toilet during the night. In industrialised society, wild animals and hostile tribes no longer pose a threat. The threat you may experience now is different. You no longer have to fight or flee, but the stress reaction you get from a deadline or other worries probably still corresponds to the stress reaction of prehistoric times: the wild animals of that time are equal to the possible stressful social or work-related circumstances of today. This stress response has a clear function. It prepares for danger and helps protect you from becoming easy prey. The bodily response to these types of contemporary stressors is probably the same as the response we showed when seeing the sabre-toothed tigers and bears of old. How can insomnia persist if the original stressful situation is no longer present? Why do our bodies not simply return to rest?

Neurologist and specialist in sleep medicine Arthur Spielman and clinical psychologist Paul Glovinsky developed a model to explain the persistent existence of insomnia. This model is largely consistent with evolutionary explanations for sleep problems. Namely, it combines:

- the predisposing factors of insomnia (what type of sleeper you are by nature) with
- the precipitating factors, such as stress from losing your job.

As long as there are no precipitating factors, a predisposition to a poor night's rest does not always lead directly to the development of long-term insomnia.

In stressful or emotional circumstances, however, insomnia can occur. Today's hunter-gatherers know virtually no long-term insomnia, and primal man probably didn't either, so why do we suffer from it? In prehistoric times, light sleepers were probably better at going back to sleep after acute danger had passed. In modern humans, another factor keeps our bodies in an alert state. Often it seems that the sleep problem itself causes this alertness, as is also described in Spielman and Glovinsky's model:

- maintaining factors: people with insomnia form certain patterns of thinking and behaviour that maintain the sleep problem after it arises.

These are the behavioural or cognitive patterns such as fretting about lying awake, napping during the day and lying in bed for long periods. We also try to control our sleep as much as possible, for example, by constantly checking what time it is and sometimes having sky-high expectations about sleeping continuously. This leads to less restful wake.[6]

An example of a negative thought people with insomnia often have is: 'If I don't sleep well, I won't be productive tomorrow.' When you think about an unpleasant event, your brain reacts as if that unpleasant event is actually happening.[7] Thus, if you think that because of poor sleep you probably will not get your work done, your brain reacts as if you are actually already in that situation. This leads to stress during the day and during the night, which in turn leads to an increase in insomnia.

In evolutionary terms, thinking of a predator causes the body to react as if the predator were actually present. Research on the role of fearful thoughts indeed suggests that these activate brain regions which reflect hypervigilance, that is: being highly alert to potential threats.[8] Therefore it is not surprising that worries keep you awake longer and lead to an increase in restless nights. After all, anxiety makes the brain want to check even more whether the environment is safe. This is supported by research showing that rumination is directly related to greater difficulty falling asleep.[9]

This may also partly explain why insomnia is more common in women. In fact, it appears that men and women handle stress differently. Women ruminate more when stressful situations arise.[10] Men are more likely to show reckless or aggressive behaviour at such times.[11] Even at the brain level, a clear gender difference can be observed after experiencing a stressful situation. More specifically, in 2007 Jiongjiong Wang and colleagues asked participants in an experiment to perform an arithmetic task in which they were prompted every 2 minutes to be faster in their performance. The researchers also asked the participants to restart the task if an error occurred. Specific parts of the brain (the anterior and posterior cingulate cortex) were activated longer in women after this stressful experiment. These brain regions are important in emotions and, according to the scientists, this might reflect a greater degree of ruminative thinking.[12] The absence of external distractions when you are lying in bed in the dark makes dealing with fretting at night even more difficult; and an overactive brain, in turn, can lead to more restless nights.

I have only talked about negative stress so far, but your sleep can also suffer from too much excitement as well – sometimes referred to as positive stress. Perhaps you recognise the situation of when you slept poorly as a child because the next day was your birthday and you expected many presents. That is an example of the way in which excitement can keep you awake and become the predator of a restful night. A fun but very busy job, or the anticipation you feel before you go on vacation, might make you too alert to doze off and keep your brain overly active. This is in line with a theory in which doing cognitive tasks can lead to being more mentally active, which can disturb our night's rest. Just having a busy mind can delay the onset of sleep, and excitement often goes together with a busy mind.[13]

Sleep reactivity

One of the predisposing factors that has gained a lot of attention in the scholarly community over the last couple of years is *sleep reactivity*. Research suggests that people with insomnia show an overly cognitive–emotional reactivity to stress, which means that they are more stressed by stress.[14] This stress dysregulation is often already present before the onset of insomnia.[15] Sleep reactivity is a concept describing the degree to which this stress translates to sleep difficulties.[16]

Various researchers have examined this characteristic by exposing people to stressful situations and measuring whether this has an influence on their sleep structure. For instance, by objectively measuring sleep, they have concluded that caffeine use and circadian shifts have variable effects. The researchers administered 400 mg of caffeine (the equivalent of 4 cups of filter coffee) to participants 30 minutes before bedtime. On other nights, the participants were asked to go to bed 3 to 6 hours before their usual bedtime. They found that some slept worse while others had an unaffected slumber, and that using too much caffeine too late and going to bed earlier than usual can indeed induce sleeplessness.[17] Other scientists tried to examine if sleep reactivity was indeed predictive of insomnia over time. They followed over 1,400 individuals during a period of 2 years and concluded that good sleepers with high sleep reactivity had a higher risk of developing insomnia.[18]

Are you born with high sleep reactivity? Twin studies show that 29–37 per cent of a person's reactivity is inheritable.[19,20] As I discussed in Chapter 1, and earlier in this chapter, sensitivity to light sleep might have helped primordial people to survive, as light sleepers were probably better at reacting to possible danger in the night. The fact that sleep reactivity is partially inheritable supports this view.

Natural selection might have induced the passing on of these 'light sleep' genes from one generation to another.

Still, genetic variability cannot explain a large percentage of this trait-like characteristic. Indeed, evidence suggests that a low baseline level can change to a higher sleep reactivity when someone experiences insomnia. Sleep system sensitisation is another word for this phenomenon.[21]

Exposure to major life events can exacerbate this effect. Several studies suggest that childhood abuse or other traumatic events increases vulnerability to insomnia as an adult. For example, one study indicated that higher incidence of childhood emotional and physical abuse correlated to more insomnia complaints during the COVID-19 pandemic, which was associated with greater sleep reactivity. In 2022 Anthony Reffi and colleagues examined 241 subjects by using questionnaires on childhood trauma and sleep and concluded that childhood abuse can lead to sleep system sensitisation.[22]

In Chapter 5, I explain that some gold standard treatment options that work in most people with insomnia often do not seem to have an effect with people who have past traumatic experiences. It seems that the scars that childhood trauma leaves in the sleep system create a high vulnerability towards sleeplessness and restless wake, and require a different approach. This is also in line with a study by Kyunga Park and colleagues at Sungshin University suggesting that people with insomnia and high sleep reactivity respond to cognitive behavioural treatment (described in Chapter 9) but show less benefit from this treatment than patients with low reactivity.[23] When people with high sleep reactivity receive treatment for their insomnia early after its onset, this might show the best results. One study showed that when people with acute insomnia (insomnia occurring for less than 3 months) received cognitive behavioural treatment at an early stage, this clearly reduced sleep reactivity and the chances of developing chronic insomnia.[24]

Are there specific characteristics in the brain of people with a sensitivity to sleep problems? As I mentioned in Chapter 2, research shows that fragmentation of REM sleep, as measured by polysomnography, may predispose some people to developing insomnia. Researchers found that traumatic and potentially traumatic events in childhood led to objectively measured fragmented sleep in children and adults, even before possible subjective insomnia emerged.[25,26] It was striking that, in the adults, these differences in REM sleep fragmentation were not related to subjective sleep quality, while a number of studies do show that people with insomnia have increased fragmentation of REM sleep. This would argue for a predisposing characteristic that is present in our brain before insomnia manifests itself. Other evidence that might support this is that sleep restriction therapy leads to a strong improvement in subjective sleep but shows no major effects on REM sleep fragmentation.[27] That makes sense, because a treatment can remove the *perpetuating* factors, but has no effect on the *predisposing* factors. It would be interesting to further investigate whether REM sleep fragmentation is indeed a biological reflection of sleep reactivity. Hopefully future studies will shed more light on this.

Mental health

While sleep reactivity is a predisposing factor for insomnia, poor mental health in general often precipitates sleeplessness. However, although insomnia is often associated with mental health problems, this is not always the case. I studied more than 200 people with insomnia in a sleep centre: it turned out that about half of all participants had no additional psychological problems.[28] In many cases, long-term insomnia presents as an isolated problem.

It is not in fact surprising that about half the participants had an anxiety disorder, depression or other psychological problem: having poor mental health can be a precipitating or a perpetuating factor for insomnia. When we fret a lot due to depression or an anxiety disorder it leads to a more hyperactive brain, and hyperactivity and sleep (or restful wake during the night) are two things that do not go well together. In addition, as discussed earlier, the behaviour of people experiencing depression sometimes creates longer-lasting symptoms of insomnia because they often stay in bed longer. This can reduce sleep pressure and lead to more problems in initiating and maintaining sleep.

However, this does not mean that insomnia with additional mental health issues is not treatable. Instead, the insomnia treatment of patients with psychiatric comorbidity can help create a more restful sleep and it can even enhance the results of the treatment of comorbid psychological problems.[29,30]

Next to mental health conditions, researchers often focus on personality traits or problems. Historically, sleep problems have been associated with perfectionism, dissatisfaction, demanding behaviours, lowered self-confidence, and high susceptibility to stress and tension.[31] Are these claims true? In my PhD study, I compared the scientific data on this topic. The problem with most scientific articles is that no clear distinction is made between insomniacs with and without additional psychiatric symptoms.[32] This is important because mental health symptoms are themselves often associated with personality traits such as high-stress sensitivity and a reduced ability to adapt one's behaviour to changing circumstances. One study indicated that personality traits of insomniacs 'normalised' when patients with additional mental health conditions were not included in the analyses.[33]

I decided to examine this phenomenon myself and found that people with insomnia, but without additional psychiatric problems, showed no specific personality traits.[34] A reason for this might be that the expression of insomnia is something that has to do with many factors, which is why people with different personality types can develop the disorder. For example, one person starts to sleep worse because of worries and being self-demanding, while another has problems keeping a regular sleep schedule because of motivational problems. The expression of the sleeplessness might be the same, but the cause might be very different and related to various personality traits.

In sum, insomnia can have many different causes. Stress, life events, genetics, mood and mental health conditions can all have a negative effect on our night's rest. However, behaviour and thoughts around sleep itself can perpetuate the sleep problem and lead to increased restlessness during the night. In the next chapter, I will describe the basic strategies to reduce these perpetuating factors of insomnia and experience a good night's rest again.

5.

The Primal Basics

'Before you go to bed, a view of the starry sky and an ear full
of music is better than any sleep aid'[1]

Hermann Hesse, *The Glass Bead Game* (1943)

While our environments have changed rapidly over the last several
hundred years, our bodies have been slower to adapt. So, what are
the primal basics – the ancient natural environmental factors that
might still have a positive influence on our sleep?

After becoming knowledgeable about sleep, it is important to
improve *sleep hygiene*. This is not (only) about changing your
sheets regularly. It is a general term that refers to behaviours and
conditions that help create a better night's rest. We do not know
much about the sleep hygiene practices of ancient cave dwellers.
What we do know is that there were no mobile devices to keep
them awake. They also had no alarm clocks to look at when being
awake at night. However, I can imagine that sleeping in a group
was sometimes a challenge. A greater chance of someone snoring
around you will certainly have had an effect on the night's rest. In
modern hunter-gatherers we know that it can still be a busy
sleeping environment at night. In the Hadza tribe in Tanzania,
married couples sleep together with their children, usually on the
same bed.[2] The ancient Greeks showed some interest in creating
optimal circumstances around the night's rest. For instance, the
Greek physician Hippocrates, who was born around 450 BCE,

recommended taking a long walk if you could not sleep.[3] I will explain why that still is a good idea!

Bed time

Can you stay in bed for too short or too long a time? Does your night's rest suffer if you go against your biological clock? If your total bed time (time spent in bed) is too short, this will often have a negative effect on your daytime functioning. This is evident from experiments in which normal sleepers were allowed to lie in bed for no more than 3–5 hours or even, in extreme cases, kept awake for a few days. The studies showed that, in general, they started to suffer from sleepiness, reduced concentration and reduced mood.[4,5]

The varying sensitivity to possible negative effects of shorter total bed times is hereditary.[6] Age also plays a role. Older people are generally less sensitive to shorter total bed times. However, there is a difference between objective and subjective measures of sleepiness. Objectively speaking, there is less sleepiness in older adults, but in their own experience, they are just as sleepy after a short night as the young.[7] Staying in bed for too short a time can also have other negative effects. More unforeseen incidents and accidents occur due to excessive sleepiness. More specifically, occupational incidents were 2½ times more likely to occur in construction workers who were overly sleepy.[8]

Depriving yourself of sleep might not be good for your daytime functioning, but as I discussed in Chapter 2, for insomniacs staying in bed too long might also have a negative effect by creating more fragmented sleep, leading to longer periods of restless wake. Indeed, in several experiments, when subjects spent longer than usual times in bed, they woke up more frequently. Sleep becomes 'saturated'. This becomes clear when you keep on staying in the bed for a longer period. Experimental studies concluded that this can lead to more fragmented sleep.[9,10] As I mentioned, this fragmented sleep does not have to be a problem, but it can become one if it leads to periods of restless wake, as is often the case in insomnia.

A good example of the effect of longer total bed time on sleep is a study that was conducted during the COVID-19 lockdowns. People slept slightly longer during this period, but the sleep became more fragmented and began to look more like Hadza sleep.[11,12,13] There are additional effects that might occur when staying in the bed for too long. Longer total bed times during the COVID-19 lockdowns may also have led to increased dream recall. Scientists concluded that frequent awakenings because of total bed time might be the reason for this. As I discussed in Chapter 3, you only remember a dream when you wake up directly from REM sleep and mostly forget it quickly. Extending total bed time often leads to more REM sleep and fragmented sleep. Simply put, waking up more often from a dream might give more opportunity to remember the dream.[14]

The length of bed time obviously influences fragmentation of sleep and subsequent daytime functioning, but how do varying total bed times affect the subjective quality of sleep? As I discussed in Chapter 1, hunter-gatherers have a very constant rhythm when it comes to activity, rest and total bed time. In industrialised societies, shift work can obviously disturb a regular day–night rhythm. What are the specific effects of shift work on our sleep? A recent study showed that it leads to shorter sleep, lying awake in bed longer and waking up more often.[15] A large systematic review found that 20–30 per cent of shift workers experience both insomnia and excessive daytime sleepiness.[16] These are signs of a condition which is called 'shift work disorder'. Older people and those who experience more morningness appear to suffer more from the negative effects of shift work on sleep, and function less well during the day. Higher eveningness is generally associated with fewer negative effects on subjective sleep quality. However, pronounced evening people logically have poorer subjective sleep quality during a period with early shifts.[17]

For people showing more morningness, it can help to get some sleep prior to the night shift. With people who show more eveningness, this is often a bit more difficult to manage, because their natural circadian rhythm leads to less sleepiness in the evening. The same may apply to people who have difficulty sleeping on a plane yet fly at night. In that case, morning people can often more easily take a long nap in the evening.

When sleeping during the day, you can expect to have less shut-eye than when sleeping at night. Adjusting expectations is therefore important. Still expecting to get your regular 6 or 7 hours of sleep can be frustrating. Therefore, it is better to focus on improving your subjective sleep quality. In the morning light, it might help to put on sunglasses when driving home after your night shift, so that your melatonin production can get going properly. Just make sure you do not get sleepy at the wheel to avoid dangerous situations. As for nutrition, it is better to take light meals at night and avoid going for that fatty snack.

With nine-to-five jobs, evening types often have the most difficulty maintaining a fixed sleep rhythm. There is a big difference between total bed times during the week and at the weekend, also known as 'social jet lag'. Students and workers compensate for too-short nights during the week by sleeping in longer at the weekend. This has the most negative consequences for subjective sleep quality in young people aged 14–25.[18]

In adults who are more evening types, sleeping in at the weekend can sometimes have advantages and lead to more energy in the morning. In one study, the subjects felt more rested if they went to bed later, got up later and slept longer. The researchers did not mention it explicitly, but social jet lag may play a role here. Normal sleepers who are more evening people sometimes deprive themselves of sleep during the week because the alarm clock goes off too early in relation to their biological clock. If they go to bed later at the weekend and get up later, they hypothetically have a day–night rhythm that better suits their biological clock and, due to a slightly longer sleep, they have less residual sleep pressure in the morning, making them more alert.[19]

So here, we are talking about average sleepers. Although it might sound like a treat, for people with insomnia sleeping in is still not a good idea because it can lead to more fragmented sleep (and subsequently less restful wake), and more problems in daytime functioning. In that case, the advantages of sleeping in often do not outweigh the disadvantages.

A good nap?

We do not know whether primordial humans napped, but as I mentioned earlier, napping is quite common in modern hunter-gatherers such as the Hadza. On average, they nap on just over half of the days of the week and napping leads to an average of 17 minutes of extra sleep per day.[20] There seems to be some uncertainty as to whether a nap is good or bad for you. As I mentioned earlier, there is a 'bright side' to napping but it depends whether you are suffering from insomnia or not.

The evidence seems to show that a short nap or a power nap during the day can have positive effects on cognitive skills. This is especially true for people who have had short total bed time the night(s) before (or sleep deprivation). In some cases, a nap can also help after a normal night.[21] For example, it can support memory and thus improve learning.[22] A power nap can also increase problem-solving skills, especially for simpler tasks.[23] For night-shift workers, sleeping briefly during a shift can help them stay alert after they wake and support their cognitive skills.[24] A nap would also make athletes more alert and it would generally not have a negative effect on physical performance. After sleep deprivation, a daytime nap can even lead to better physical performance.[25]

How to nap? If you take a short nap, it is good not to make it longer than 30 minutes, otherwise you may suffer from sleep inertia afterwards – the increased sleepiness that can occur directly after waking up and which can last for a while. Napping longer is only recommended if you spent too little time in bed the night(s) before. In that case, you can nap for 90 minutes. After that period, most people have pretty much gone through an entire sleep cycle and you might wake up more pleasantly. Shorter napping (30–60 minutes) after a late night does not seem to be sufficient to compensate for the negative cognitive effects of sleep deprivation.[26]

The timing and frequency of the nap also seems to be important. Napping more than three times a week and napping for more than 2 hours at a time is associated with poorer subjective sleep quality. Napping too late (for example between 6 p.m. and 9 p.m.) is associated with a shorter night sleep.[27] Can napping really trigger chronic insomnia? There appears to be a difference between indiscriminate nappers and people who have incorporated napping into a fixed pattern in their lives. The first group is three times more likely to develop chronic insomnia.[28] For people who incorporate the nap as a pattern into their daily lives, the chance is about 1.5 times bigger instead of 3. Why the difference? People who nap haphazardly are more likely to use this sleep period to compensate for bad nights than the other group.

Is it wise to nap if you already suffer from insomnia? It turns out that taking naps when you already suffer from insomnia can be counterproductive. The same as with sleeping in, when you are a bad sleeper it is better not to nap. It is of course logical that after a number of bad nights you might be happy with some extra sleep, even if it is during the day. However, people who have been sleeping poorly for a longer time and who nap more often, lie awake longer during the night and, in the case of insomnia, this is usually not a restful night-time wake period.[29,30]

Last year I read a newspaper article in which the reporter stated that napping would lead to an early death. With such news items, it is always important to look at the original source. The reporter referred to a study by Ming-Jing Yang and colleagues in which frequency of napping appeared to be associated with hypertension and stroke. However, an association or correlation is not yet a causal relationship, which the researchers clearly stated in their study.[31] An explanation might be that underlying somatic problems both cause hypertension or stroke, but also lead to more napping. An example of such a somatic problem could be sleep apnoea. More specifically, sleep apnoea might result in excessive daytime sleepiness, which might lead to increased napping, and, as mentioned earlier, sleep apnoea can increase the risk of cardiovascular problems. Apart from the fact that napping a lot during the day is usually not a good idea, the claim that napping would lead to an early death was yet another example of bad journalism, which can plague the sleep world.

You snooze, you lose

Cave dwellers obviously could not make use of a snooze button in the mornings. They were probably able to follow their own biological clock more, meaning they were less abruptly woken up from sleep by an alarm clock. You can imagine that this is much more natural and might lead to more stable circadian rhythms, as it does for contemporary hunter-gatherers. Unfortunately waking up at a natural time is no longer an option for many people these days, due to work obligations. Nowadays, slapping the snooze button is common practice.

In a survey examining 20,000 users of activity-tracking wristwatches, 50 per cent of people admitted they use the snooze button at least once every morning. What are the effects of snoozing?

A 2022 Japanese study showed that more than 70 per cent of people snoozed, mainly to reduce anxiety because of possible oversleeping. The researchers used polysomnography to quantify sleep. During the last 20 minutes of sleep, snoozing prolonged wake and NREM1 (light) sleep. The objective quality of sleep was therefore poorer for the snoozers. Another finding was that they had a longer period of sleep inertia in the morning compared to people who use a single alarm. In other words, the transition of sleep to wake took more time, leaving the snoozers drowsier in the morning.[32] A possible reason for this is that transitions into and from sleep induce changes in the body that might inhibit smooth awakenings. For example, your heart rate increases when waking up and your body constantly has to perform kickstarts through every awakening. This costs energy and might leave a person more tired and sleepy in the morning after snoozing.[33]

As mentioned earlier, sleep inertia might have a positive effect on sleep, especially during episodes of wakefulness in the night. Drowsiness in nightly awakenings might protect our sleep and increase the drive to fall asleep again.[34] Therefore the repeated forced awakenings in the morning because of a snooze alarm might lead to a higher threshold of awakening because the body wants to protect sleep, which could lead to more sleepiness in snoozers.

A 2023 study showed somewhat different results. These scientists concluded that snoozing has a positive effect on the performance of a cognitive task and does not affect sleepiness in the morning.[35]

How can we explain the difference between the study results? The first study only used auditory reaction times and a 10-point scale to assess alertness, sleepiness, motivation loss, weariness and cognitive functioning after awakening. The researchers in 2023, who found a positive effect on snoozing, used cognitive tests that were more demanding for the participants, measuring aspects such as arithmetic speed and episodic memory. Possibly, regular snoozers might benefit from snoozing if they have to perform slightly more complex tasks after waking up. A more negative finding was that the snoozers experienced more sleepiness during the day and had to use more effort later in the day to perform cognitive tasks.

In summary, although the evidence of a positive or negative effect of snoozing on sleep inertia and cognitive functioning in the morning is mixed, the general advice is to try to stop snoozing and get out of the bed after a single alarm. Although it might benefit more complex cognitive functioning just after waking up in regular snoozers, it might also have a negative effect on the rest of your day, leading to sleepiness and more needed effort to get you through the day.

Shedding some light

Compared to prehistoric humans, we modern humans experience far longer light exposure, especially during evening and night, which has to do with the use of artificial light. Light is important for sleep quality and the proper functioning of our biological clock. That clock is set to a natural environment and not to the fluorescent beams of that fast-food store where you go to grab a late-night snack. The presumption is that light in the evening keeps you awake. Sufficient morning light would actually be good for your circadian rhythm. What does science say about this? Does light affect sleep?

In the Hadza tribe, Samson found that the amount of light that study participants were exposed to when they were out of bed was related to the length of sleep.[36] The more light, the shorter the sleep, and that is not a surprise.

You can imagine that with the advent of artificial light, people have become exposed to light for much longer. However, because people in industrialised societies often spend less time outdoors, the amount of light we get during the day is probably a lot less. What effect could that have on our sleep?

Almost all light has an effect on sleep quality and on our circadian rhythm, but in most cases the light intensity, or *lux*, is especially important: 1 lux equals the light of 1 candle that is 1 metre away. The ratio between the amount of light during the day and the evening is decisive. I will tell you more about that later. To give you an idea of this measure of light intensity: bright daylight is approximately 10,000 lux, an overcast day is 1,000 lux, while a well-lit office sometimes only just reaches 500 lux. The wavelength is another factor when looking at light.

You may have heard that exposure to blue light from lamps or device screens just before bed has the worst effect on sleep quality and timing, but there's a catch. Many studies have been conducted on blue light and sleep, but most of these studies were poorly designed.[37] An example of this is a study performed in 2009 in the US with people with insomnia. It appears that this group slept slightly better after wearing 'blue light filter' glasses.[38] Unfortunately, the sample size was very small (20 people) and there were other problems with the study design, making it difficult to draw conclusions. Another study in 2018 produced similar results, but again few test subjects (14) were included.[39] A major systematic review took place in 2021.[40] The conclusion was that the evidence for a positive effect of blue light filtering on subjective sleep quality is very weak and contradictory. Some glasses, such as those with orange, well-sealed lenses, seem to filter out more blue light than others. However, the effect of these glasses on sleep quality also seems to be limited. Young people who wear orange glasses before sleeping may have significantly better subjective sleep quality, but the difference in sleep quality itself was very small.[41]

It is not surprising that filtering out blue light seems to have a limited effect on sleep quality. It turns out that light of other wavelengths (determining the colour you perceive) can also lead to changes in your sleep.[42] In general, it is not so much the wavelength, but rather the amount of light that is important (and its distribution over the day) for sleep quality. In contrast, for the timing of your sleep, blue light in the evening might have a negative effect, pushing the biological clock backwards. However, when the amount of light is low enough, the colour of the light is generally less important for our biological clocks.

Can you use screens before going to bed or not? Moreover, are smartphones messing up our sleep quality and circadian rhythm? Indeed, longer smartphone use is associated with poorer sleep.[43] The only question is: is this because of the light? In the past, scientists often stated that smartphones affect our melatonin balance, which disrupts our circadian rhythms and more specifically the onset of sleep. More recent research has indicated that smartphones do not have much effect on melatonin at all.[44] Apparently, there is another reason why people sleep worse after use their smartphones, which I will come back to.

Although a smartphone probably does not emit enough light to disrupt your sleep, it seems to be a different story when looking at computers and iPads, because they emit more light. It is important how long you use such a screen. Researchers state that use of an iPad on the brightest setting 2 hours before trying to sleep clearly suppresses melatonin.[45] Still, it is not only the light from the iPad, but also what you do on your screen that can disrupt sleep. For example, the night mode of your iPad provides minimal protection against the negative effects of screen use.[46] 'Active' screens before bed are not a good idea, not so much because of light exposure, but rather because of the brain activity it usually requires. In computers or iPads, the light could play a role after prolonged exposure. In line with this, it turns out that watching TV has less effect on sleep than smartphone, iPad or computer use.[47] Watching a TV programme or movie is usually a more passive form of media use, making you less alert than with other devices. Being less alert in the evening helps with better sleep. In a theoretical review in 2024, researcher Serena Bauducco concluded that there might be a bi-directional link between the use of technology and sleep problems and that media use might not only create sleep problems but sometimes also be used as a time filler or a strategy to regulate emotions, which can actually help people to sleep better. According to Bauducco, removing technology from bedrooms overnight might help some, but in others removing it might not be helpful because it could lead to more negative thoughts and arousal which might hamper sleep. It is important to find out what works for you and there is no one size fits all.[48]

What is the best amount of ambient light to use during the day and night? A recent recommendation from experts in this field answers this question:

Optimal light in the morning and during the day

Timing of light is important for sleep quality. A study from the Netherlands concluded that later exposure to a light intensity similar to morning twilight is associated with waking up more often and staying awake for longer.[49] Therefore, exposing yourself to enough bright light early in the morning seems like a good idea, because it may help you sleep better the next night.

According to experts, you should have at least 250 lux during the day to maintain a good circadian rhythm.[50] They do not use the normal light measure, but the 'melanopic equivalent daylight illuminance' (mEDI) which takes the wavelength of light into account. Huh? Wavelength of light was not that important for quality and timing of sleep, was it? Well, not in normal circumstances, because then you naturally get enough light during the day (such as outside or under a stronger lamp). In the evening you get substantially less light and at low light intensities the colour of the light has less impact on our sleep timing and quality. However, if you stay in a badly lit office during the day and expose yourself to too much light (outside) in the evening, the colour of the light definitely has an influence on your biological clock. You can compare a mEDI of 250 lux to a sufficiently 'coolly lit' office. The lighting or outside light ensures that you can do your work well. But this is a minimum, because more is better! Next to a positive influence on your circadian rhythm, intensive ambient light during the day can also lead to better sleep quality.[51] Test subjects literally slept more deeply after exposure to intense light during the 'awake' intervals.

If you expose yourself primarily to artificial (and probably warmer and weaker) light during the day, you appear to be more sensitive to the negative effects of light in the evening. If you have been outside a lot during the day, this protects against the negative effects of evening light and promotes a good sleep.[52] In other words: a walk outside during the day can have a positive effect on your sleep quality and timing. A side note regarding the possible causal relationship in this study is that people who work indoors may undertake less physical exercise and this may play a role in the results. Nevertheless, if that were the case, walking (outside) would still be a good idea! Another article showed that plenty of light during the day can reduce the negative effects of screen use in the evening.[53] But of course, the rule still applies: don't be too active on your screen before bed.

Optimal light during the evening

During the evening, it is important to dim the lights as much as possible. The less light you have had during the day, the more this can help. Experts mention a recommended maximum mEDI of

10 lux, starting 3 hours before you go to bed.[54] This is comparable to evening twilight. In short: turn off those fluorescent beams in the evening and use as little light as possible in the last hours before you go to bed: think of light from a weak table lamp that is reminiscent of a candle in terms of warmth and that is sufficiently far away from you. Could you make it even darker during those evening hours? For example, some people only have the TV on in the evening in the dark, and from a sleep point of view, that might not be a bad idea at all.

Optimal light at night

At night, the light intensity should not exceed a mEDI of 1 lux, which is extremely dark. A negative effect on our objective sleep quality can already occur at very low light intensities at night. Even if you close your eyes, very dim light can affect your sleep.[55]

In a nutshell, most light affects sleep quality and timing. Badly timed exposure to too much or too little light can have a negative effect on your objective and subjective sleep quality. Filtering blue light does not seem to help much to improve sleep quality. Furthermore, under normal circumstances, for our biological clocks, the wavelength of light seems less important than the amount of light. It is better to put away 'active' screens, such as smartphones and computers, just before going to bed, particularly because of what you do on that screen. 'Passive' screens such as TVs have less effect on sleep. Exposing yourself to enough light early in the morning seems to be a good thing. In addition, go outside during the day! It is likely to make you less sensitive to light exposure in the evening and can support your sleep quality. When you have had little light exposure during the day, it is extra important to dim the lights in the evening 3 hours before you go to bed. Do you think your living room already looks like a basement in an eighties horror movie? Then make it even darker. At night, it is best to have a pitch-black bedroom. What can help is to wear a sleeping mask at night or, for example, to ask the neighbours to turn off the garden lighting if it shines through the gaps in the blackout curtains.

Seasonal variations

In March every year the clocks are set forward by one hour in approximately 70 countries. The idea of this daylight saving time is that it helps to make optimal use of daylight because in spring, summer and early autumn it gets dark later. Advocates of daylight saving time indicate that this would lead to less use of electrical light, which might be good for environmental and economic purposes. In 2020, the American Academy of Sleep Medicine stated that governments should abolish seasonal time changes because it might lead to circadian misalignment and negative health effects.[56]

Our primordial ancestors probably determined the time from natural variations in light and temperature, and a precise clock was not available. Temperature might be a more important game-changer than light when it comes to living conditions between summer and winter. There is evidence that prehistoric humans migrated between summer and winter camps to make full use of natural resources in some parts of the world. Summer camps would be at high altitude and winter camps at low altitude. One study indicates that for a group of cave dwellers in Tibet, travelling time would have been less than 45 days between their two camps.[57]

We cannot examine if there were differences between sleep in winter and sleep in summer in prehistoric man but studies in contemporary hunter-gatherers suggest that this might have been the case. Scientists found that sleep duration, as measured by actigraphy, decreases from winter to summer: in summer, hunter-gatherers go to bed later and sleep an hour less. In addition, napping occurs three times as often in the summer. This usually takes place during the afternoon, in the shade, out of the heat of the day.[58]

In industrialised societies, there is also an observed seasonal variation in sleep. We, like the contemporary hunter-gatherers, generally have a shorter night's rest in the summer and longer in the winter.[59] In contrast with today's hunter-gatherers, people from industrialised societies typically report longer sleep in winter because of later wake times rather than earlier sleep times.[60] Probably this difference has to do with artificial lighting and our climate-controlled environments, which expose our bodies to fewer natural variations in light and temperature. In winter, we can put the heating on in the evening and expose ourselves longer to light, which possibly diminishes the effects this season would naturally have had on our sleep. This would explain why seasonal variations in sleep duration are smaller in industrialised societies than in contemporary hunter-gatherers. Instead of an hour shorter sleep in summer, one study found a difference of 12 minutes when compared to winter.[61]

As I indicated earlier, light often has a major effect on our day–night rhythms, and depending on the latitude at which you live, seasonal variation in light exposure might have a greater impact on your sleep. In countries far from the Equator, such as Iceland, light conditions around sleep vary greatly across the seasons. That is why in most of these countries extra attention is paid to making the bedroom dark, while at other times the focus is on using bright-light lamps to create a better day–night rhythm.

Hot stuff

In addition to light, adequate ambient temperature is an important factor in maintaining good sleep. In Chapter 1, I mentioned that today's hunter-gatherers show circadian rhythms adapted to the temperature of their environment. An ambient temperature drop is a signal for your biological clock that bedtime is approaching. Research has indicated that individuals who are satisfied with the temperature of their environment experience better sleep quality.[62]

Body temperature is also very important in sleep. Usually this is around 37 degrees Celsius (98.6 degrees Fahrenheit) but during the night this can go down by 1 degree Celsius (1.8 degrees Fahrenheit).[63] Two hours before falling asleep, our core body temperature starts to decrease.[64] In general, the bigger the reduction in core body temperature, the shorter time you need to fall asleep.[65] Two hours before waking up, our core body temperatures start to rise again.

If our core body temperature decreases, heat usually transmits through the skin that is furthest away from the core. This means that the blood vessels in body parts like our hands and feet will need to dilate in order to lose heat, which makes them feel warm.[66] This is a reason why many people cannot fall asleep when their hands or feet are cold. They are simply unable to lose enough heat to fall asleep. Therefore, it is not surprising that chronic cold feet are associated with sleep-onset insomnia.[67] Sometimes bed socks can help, warming up the feet so we can fall asleep more easily.

Of course, to create a body temperature drop before going to bed, you do not have to freeze. However, do be aware of the ambient temperature at night and throw out that extra warm layer.[68] Another tip is to take a hot shower, bath or to exercise a few hours before you go to sleep. The temperature of the body increases and, once you finish, you naturally cool down just before going to bed.[69]

How hot should your bedroom be? The ideal bedroom temperature is somewhere between 15.5 and 20.5 degrees Celsius (60–69 degrees Fahrenheit). Furthermore, the temperature under your bedding should be between 27 and 31 degrees Celsius (80–88 degrees Fahrenheit) to create a good sleep environment.[70,71] Women are usually more comfortable with a slightly higher temperature in the bed than men.[72] It is important to create a sleep environment that is cool enough, because the regulation of body temperature can decrease during our sleep. Specifically, during REM sleep, there is less regulation of body heat, such as sweating or shivering. This makes a person more sensitive to ambient heat.[73] High temperatures in the night are uncomfortable and can disrupt objective sleep quality. For instance, there is a link between higher body temperature during sleep and a lower amount of deep and REM sleep.[74] Also, scientists found, people living in hotter climates generally sleep for a shorter amount of time, with night-time outside temperatures above 10 degrees Celsius (50 degrees Fahrenheit) being associated with a shorter night's rest.[75]

A way of counteracting heat is to use air conditioning. Some experts advise using air conditioning in the bedroom while others advise against it. What does science say? According to a 2015 study by Japanese researchers, the use of air conditioning can lead to more frequent awakenings, especially if, for instance, it is aimed directly at the body. They therefore advise to set up an air conditioner in such a way that it does not direct a strong airflow towards the body.[76] On the other hand, it is also important not to be too cold at night. In a study of the Hadza tribe, it was found that warmer temperatures were associated with longer sleep. Researchers concluded that this probably has to do with the fact that the Hadza can suffer more from cold at night and that warmer temperatures at night therefore lead to more sleeping comfort.[77]

Recently, I read a newspaper article stating that due to rising ambient temperatures it is predicted we will sleep 44 hours less every year. I decided to examine the original study. In the summary, Kelton Minor and colleagues clearly indicated that rising temperatures might amount to an average of 50–58 hours less sleep in 2099 when compared to 2022.[78] According to my calculations, we would then sleep an average of 0.75 hours (45 minutes) less per year, not 44 hours, which is a bit of a relief. A recent review article indicated that studies on rising ambient temperatures from climate change are scarce, so to draw clear conclusions on this topic, we need more research.[79]

Modern straw beds

We know that prehistoric humans slept on beds of straw, branches and leaves, but nowadays most people use mattresses and more comfortable materials. What influence do these modern beds have on our night's rest?

As discussed earlier, body heat regulation is an important part of the cyclical structure of our sleep. Therefore, materials that support thermoregulation might be beneficial. Many people will recognise the experience that a bed that feels too warm can negatively influence your sleep. What does science say about this? Indeed, a lot of research in recent years shows a connection between bed materials and subjective and objective sleep quality.

Certain types of mattress might have a positive effect on your objective sleep quality. Specifically, a mattress with a high thermal capacity ensures a greater drop in core temperature, which is a natural process that usually precedes sleep.[80] It's not just the mattress that you have to consider. Pillows with good thermoregulatory properties also seem to be the best choice.[81] For a good sleep it is important to keep your hands and feet warm, but your head cool.

Next to temperature, comfort is another aspect that people often look for when buying a new mattress. Nobody wants to sleep on a mattress that feels like a rock or that is so soft that you completely disappear into it. Research finds that people who rate their mattress as comfortable have a higher subjective sleep quality and objectively spend less time awake.[82] However, what is comfortable for one person does not have to be the same for the other. Nevertheless, two recent reviews showed that a medium-firm mattress is associated with better subjective sleep quality for most people.[83,84] The problem with general advice around firmness of mattresses is that there can be large differences in a person's sleeping position and body weight. People who are heavier generally need a firmer mattress to support their body. The support needed when sleeping on your back might be different from sleeping on the side or stomach. For instance, stomach sleepers often need a firmer mattress than back sleepers do. It is always good to try a mattress first, check whether it is comfortable, and whether it gives enough support. Furthermore, mattresses also have a limited lifespan. The general advice is to replace them on average every 6–8 years due to loss of comfort and support.

In terms of comfort, the same goes for pillows. A recent meta-analysis found that rubber and spring pillows perform best. Scientific data is not clear about the optimal height and shape of the pillow.[85] It makes sense that general advice for pillow height is difficult, because it also depends on what kind of sleeper you are. People sleeping on their stomach often need lower pillows than back sleepers do. A lower pillow might help relieve neck strain in stomach sleepers.

Can bedding material enhance sleep quality? Experts often advise for natural and breathable materials, though the material of bed-sheets does not appear to make a difference.[86] Weighted blankets could be supportive of sleep, but a review indicated that there are significant methodological limitations in the studies conducted.[87] A specific group that might benefit is people with mental health conditions. In this group, insomnia complaints decreased when using a weighted blanket.[88] The idea is that the weighted blankets have a positive effect on sleep because the deep pressure stimulation calms the body and brings relaxation.

What effect does the material of nightwear or pyjamas have on sleep quality? It seems that woollen fabrics might be the best for your night's rest. At an ambient temperature of 17 degrees Celsius, but also at 22 degrees Celsius (62–72 degrees Fahrenheit), woollen pyjamas perform better than cotton pyjamas, as measured by polysomnography. In short, what kind of materials you wear, sleep on or under can certainly influence your sleep quality.

Sleeping with the enemy

As this title suggests, I am going to talk about something that can really hamper your night's rest. It is also the title of a scientific article on the sleep-inhibiting effect of watching the clock during the night.[89] Many people who experience insomnia monitor the time during the night. It can create a sense of control over your sleep, but in practice this is not real control: it only makes sleep problems worse and leads to more stress in the bed. I recognise the excessive clock-watching at night from the period of my own insomnia. Knowing what time it was gave me some sense of apparent control, but I was kept awake by the thought that I could only sleep for a few more hours.

In a 2023 study, Spencer Dawson and colleagues examined sleep medication use and pre-sleep time-monitoring behaviour in almost 5,000 people. They found that watching the clock can aggravate insomnia complaints and that this might lead to the use of more sleep medication. Another explanation might be that people who experience more severe sleep problems tend to watch the clock more and use more sleep medication because of these problems.[90]

Another study gives more insight into a possible causal relationship. Thirty good and thirty bad sleepers were instructed to either watch the clock or not, when trying to fall asleep. Clock-watching was associated with a longer time needed to doze off. This was the case for bad sleepers but surprisingly held for good sleepers too. In both groups, it took the participants around 25 minutes longer to fall asleep when they were watching the clock.

What is the explanation for this phenomenon? The hypothesis is that watching the clock leads to more pre-sleep worry.[91] In turn this leads to more cognitive arousal, which can inhibit sleep. Indeed, the researchers found that pre-sleep clock-watching did increase worrying in bed. As discussed earlier, cave dwellers did not have alarm clocks to see what the time was and relied on gradual changes in ambient temperature and light. Possibly, this was a more natural way to estimate time when needed and did not lead to the control mechanism of clock-watching that many of us display nowadays when facing sleep problems.

The conclusion is that it is important to remove visible clocks from the bedroom as much as possible – some people even have a projection clock that projects the time onto the ceiling. It is important to move these as far away from your bedroom as possible and try to get through the night without a clock. The same applies to mobile phones. Many patients I saw would check their phones at night to find out what time it was. I often advised moving the phone far from the bed so that people were not tempted to look at it.

Stay active

Does exercise help you sleep better? Do top athletes sleep worse or better than the average person? Is it possible to exercise too much? Does it matter whether you do cardio or strength training? What does science say about exercise just before you go to bed? I will try to answer a few questions surrounding this topic.

First of all, there were interesting findings in the 2017 study of the Hadza tribe. On average, more activity was associated with shorter sleep.[92] The researchers did not comment further on this connection. My own thinking on an interplay here is that people who sleep shorter spend less time in bed and are simply more active because they have less total bed time. In other words: more exercise does not lead to shorter sleep, but shorter sleep leads to more exercise. Further research should of course show whether this hypothesis is correct.

A Chinese review published in 2021 shows that regular exercise leads to significantly better sleep in adults and a reduction of insomnia complaints.[93] This mainly concerns subjective improvements in symptoms, because objective sleep measurements do not show any progress. Exercise programmes have a more positive effect on middle-aged and older adults than on the younger population: the older groups clearly have better subjective sleep quality and longer sleep duration. It does not seem to matter how intensive the programme is and whether they lift weights or go for a run on a treadmill: the effects are the same. There is no difference between strength training or cardio.[94] The fact that exercise has a greater effect in the older population might have to do with the fact that they are on the whole physically less active to start with, which is why they might benefit more from exercise.

The effect of exercise on sleep quality in children, adolescents and young adults is unclear because the studies contradict each other.[95] One study showed that young people had more improvement in sleep quality when they participated in high-intensity aerobic training.[96] However, a recent systematic review describes that moderate sporting activities have a better effect on the night's rest than very intensive activities for people both young and old.[97]

Next to a positive effect on sleep, exercise before going to bed might also lead to a smoother start to the day. It seems that exercise is not only good for sleep but also for an energetic feeling when waking up. According to a 2022 study by Raphael Vallat and colleagues, if you have been more active the day before, you will wake up fitter and more alert the next morning.[98]

What is the effect of exercise on poor sleepers? Adult poor sleepers may sleep slightly better after an exercise programme.[99] The older you are, the stronger the potential (positive) effect of exercise on your sleep. Middle-aged and older poor sleepers experience better sleep quality after following a training programme. They also need less time to fall asleep and use less sleep medication.[100] The positive effects of exercise on poor sleepers are in line with the knowledge we have about basic sleep mechanisms. More specifically, in Chapter 2 I discussed the role of sleep pressure on the subjective quality of a night's rest. Shorter total bed times and more exercise stimulate this process and might lead to fewer problems initiating and maintaining sleep and shorter periods of restless wake.

In people with mental health conditions, exercise can also have a positive effect on subjective sleep quality. One study showed that people with a depressive disorder or PTSD had better sleep after an exercise programme in addition to psychological treatment than after psychological treatment alone.[101] Scientists found that in people with generalised anxiety disorder, both strength training and aerobic training had a positive influence on sleep, with a small preference for strength training. Another great result was that anxiety complaints decreased in addition to a reduction in sleep problems.[102] Exercise is not only good for mental health, but also for sleep.

In conclusion, exercise is usually good for your sleep, but what is the right time for it? Working out in the evening might make you too active to fall asleep, right?

A large meta-analysis indicated that research results on the effect of high-intensity exercise on your subjective sleep quality are mixed.[103] A systematic review shows that working out in the evening sometimes even seems to improve sleep.[104] However, you should take the time of day into account. One study indicates that it is better to stop intensive exercise 2 hours before going to bed, while according to another, it is fine to exercise up to 1 hour before going to bed. Why should you stop in good time? When you work out too late, your body does not have enough time to return to a resting state. It may then take longer for you to doze off and your sleep will be shorter.[105]

Top athletes often push their bodies to the limits and regularly participate in extreme forms of physical exercise. If you are a top athlete, are you more likely to have sleep problems? There are few known high-quality studies, but in general, elite athletes suffer more from insomnia. It takes them longer to fall asleep and they wake up more often. Over one-third and up to one-half of elite athletes are poor sleepers.[106] This is considerably more than the 20 per cent who generally describe themselves as bad sleepers in the general population.

A theory about this high prevalence is that it is not the exercise, but the fact that such athletes tend to be young and high achievers. Performance pressure probably has a negative effect on sleep. Just before a match or competition, this effect becomes even clearer. Sleep problems among top athletes often increase at that time. This increase is similar to the sleep problems in ballet dancers before a performance or in students before an exam.[107,108] A possible reason for this is that 'hyperarousal' and being too alert can prevent good sleep. You end up in too much survival mode, so to speak. Nervousness or being worried about the competition causes this alertness.[109]

In elite athletes, the type of sport matters when it comes to sleep. For example, top swimmers need an average of 40 minutes to fall asleep, while rugby players only need an average of 8 minutes.[110] Research found that there is a clear difference in the sleep patterns of team athletes and individual athletes. The latter group often reports worse sleep. The explanation for this might be that in a team there is divided responsibility for performance, which can have a lesser impact on sleep.[111]

In summary, exercise is good for your sleep. The older you get, the greater the effect of an exercise programme. This may have something to do with the fact that older people exercise less anyway. Indeed, research indicates that older people exercise less intensively and are more often inactive.[112] This means that a programme might have a positive influence more quickly. Age also appears to play a role in people with insomnia. Older poor sleepers respond better to an exercise programme.

People with mental health conditions benefit from an exercise programme in addition to psychological guidance. This can improve both sleep and psychological condition. There usually is no difference between strength training and cardio when it comes to a positive effect in sleep. Exercising in the evening is fine, but it is wise not to exercise too intensively 1 to 2 hours before going to bed; otherwise, by the time you go to bed, you simply will not be calm enough to fall asleep.

Moonstruck

It takes 29.5 days for the moon to go from full to new and back again. The cycle has eight phases in total, of which the full moon is one. In nature, there are various relationships with the nocturnal light source. For example, the thickness of tree stems and reproduction of crabs show variations based on the phase of the moon.[113,114]

There are several conflicting studies when it comes to the moon and human sleep. According to one study measuring objective sleep quality, during a full moon it takes us 5 minutes longer to doze off, we sleep 20 minutes less, we have 30 per cent less deep sleep and we also feel that we sleep worse.[115] Another study also concluded that we objectively sleep 25 minutes less and that we wake up more often in between.[116]

In contrast, after analysing several large data sets, in 2014 a team of researchers did not find a connection at all between the full moon and poorer night's rest.[117] Maren Cordi and colleagues concluded that the earlier conclusions were based on what's called a 'file-drawer problem': that scientists had looked for data to test their hypothesis in studies which had been originally used for other purposes and then filed away. If this happens often enough, there is always a high chance of a coincidental finding. Subsequently, scientists are more likely to publish something if they find a confirmation of their hypothesis than if this is not the case. The result is a publication bias.

A large 2021 study by Leandro Casiraghi and colleagues confirmed that there are no links between poor sleep, as measured by actigraphy, and the full moon, but scientists did find something else. They investigated 464 students in urban America and 98 Argentine indigenous Toba people (also known as the Qom). The test subjects appeared to doze off later and sleep shorter in the 3–5 days preceding a full moon.[118] The results were the same for both groups, regardless of access to electric lighting.

How is this possible? One fact is that the moon rises an average of 50 minutes later every day. A few days before the full moon, it is therefore at its highest point in the early evening and therefore most moonlight is present. It is thought that we have adapted our sleeping patterns to the position of the moon in such a way that we sleep less on moonlit evenings because the light allows us to be active (for example, hunting and fishing) for longer. Nice hypothesis, but that does not explain why the students in the study showed the same effect. After all, they have so much light pollution around them in the evening that it would cancel out any effect of moonlight.

The further question is whether the strength of the moonlight can contribute to falling asleep later. The light level of the full moon ranges from 0.1 to 0.25 lux. A supermoon would be a maximum of 0.32 lux. I already indicated that the light should not exceed a mEDI of 10 lux in the evening and a mEDI of 1 lux at night, so the moon level is a lot lower.[119] Nor would the light explain why people in rooms without windows also slept worse during a full moon.

The moon phase also seemed to correlate with sleep patterns in the Hadza tribe, only the effect turned out to be the opposite of what you might expect. In the Hadza, more moonlight was associated with longer sleep. The researchers indicated that one of the reasons is that the Hadza perform certain rituals on completely dark nights. An example of this is the *epeme* dance, performed when there is no moon in sight. It is believed that this ritual ensures bonding within the tribe and future success in hunting.[120]

So, in general: yes, there seems to be a connection between the moon phase and sleep, but it is unclear why. It is important that you are not too concerned with the position of the moon, however. The thought that you will not sleep well when a full moon approaches probably has more influence than the phase of the moon itself.

You sleep how you eat

Does a low-carb diet affect your night's rest? Is it true that bananas and warm milk can promote sleep? Does it matter how many carbohydrates, proteins and fats you eat?

A recent systematic review of 19 studies found that subjectively good sleepers eat more protein-rich meals than poor sleepers do.[121] Relatively speaking, good sleepers consumed 1.5 times as much protein. Poor sleepers got their energy more from carbohydrates and fats. People with poor subjective sleep quality ate up to almost 1.8 times as much fat. Unfortunately, the studies do not tell us anything about a causal relationship. For example, could it be that poor sleepers are more likely to turn to fat and carbohydrates because they feel tired?

Well, there are indications that you will actually sleep better if your diet includes more proteins.[122] In overweight people, following a higher protein diet for 4 weeks led to better subjective sleep than a diet with less protein. Another study showed that eating more protein was associated with shorter sleep.[123] How can this data be so contradictory? First of all, the latter study did not look at the percentage of proteins, but at protein intake in total. (The difficulty of this study is also a somewhat messy design, in which some of the test subjects followed a diet and some did not, and this was not controlled for; it is therefore not clear whether there are effects on sleep due to a change in the composition of carbohydrates, proteins and fats.) And it's essential to remember that sleep duration is not the same as sleep quality. Someone who sleeps shorter does not necessarily sleep worse. Overall, there appears to be more evidence for the benefits than for the disadvantages of a high-protein diet on sleep; it seems likely there is a causal relationship whereby a relatively higher protein intake leads to better sleep.

Regarding fats and carbohydrates, the data is contradictory. There has also been little experimental research measuring the effect of fat and carbohydrate intake on sleep. In general, eating less fat has been associated with better subjective sleep, but a causal relationship is unclear.[124] There is one old study involving 8 test subjects, in which eating a lot of carbohydrates and few fats led to a shortening of deep sleep.[125] In general, eating relatively fewer carbohydrates is associated with better objective sleep. The difficulty with the limited number of studies is that few test subjects are used. Furthermore, carbohydrates with a varying glycaemic index (this represents the relative ability to increase the level of glucose in the blood) are often used. As a result, the scientific conclusions can be somewhat variable.[126]

How long before going to bed should you stop eating? A recent study indicated that eating late could give you between 25 and 35 minutes longer sleep, but also poorer subjective sleep quality. People who ate a meal within an hour of going to bed stayed awake longer in between.[127] It is unclear whether eating later is related to other (un)healthy behaviours, such as keeping total bed times that are too long, which can cause late eaters to have poor subjective sleep quality. Another recent study also showed that late eaters sleep worse. Young adults who ate within 3 hours of going to bed woke up more often.[128] Again, we know nothing about causality, or whether other factors can explain this association. Nevertheless, it seems that eating too late is not conducive to good sleep.

However, feeling hungry when trying to sleep is not really helping, so if this happens, what is the best thing to eat? Eating a bag of potato chips just before going to bed does not seem to be beneficial for your sleep. If you eat a lot of carbohydrates and fats within an hour of going to bed, this can lead to objectively staying awake longer.[129] The fact that eating fatty foods late leads to poorer sleep also seems to emerge from a more recent study. Eating kebabs late at night, for example, had a negative impact on subjective sleep quality in one study.[130] (When looking at the research methods, I immediately noticed a number of variables that could influence the study results. In contrast with the other research participants, the scientists took the kebab-eating subjects to a restaurant. The question is of course whether the car ride to the restaurant at 10 p.m. and the (fluorescent?) lighting contributed to poorer sleep.)

I have mainly discussed fats, proteins and carbohydrates, but what about nutritional supplements? There is a lot of advertising about the sleep-promoting effects of nutritional supplements, but are the claims well founded? While an earlier study was somewhat more positive, a large meta-analysis from 2022 critically examined the scientific articles surrounding vitamins and nutritional supplements.[131] It found that very small studies had been conducted and the quality of research was poor. This was the case for published research into vitamin D, zinc and amino acids. In 2021, a review concluded that the effect of valerian and chamomile is highly questionable.[132] In 2023 Johanna Ell and colleagues again found a lack of strong evidence for a positive effect of valerian on sleep.[133] As far as the amino acid tryptophan is concerned, a meta-analysis concluded that it can support sleep and that people who use more than 1 milligram, in particular, sleep better.[134]

Lifestyle experts often advise taking melatonin to improve sleep. However, a 2022 meta-analysis showed that melatonin does not appear to be effective in adults. For children and adolescents with insomnia, melatonin might help them fall asleep sooner and might lead to longer sleep.[135] It can have unpleasant side effects, however: in 2023, Danish researchers found that these can include headache, nausea, skin irritation, mood swings, tiredness and dizziness.[136] Also in 2023, researchers concluded that because of its possible side effects and yet unknown possible negative effects in people with somatic disease, melatonin should be considered as a medication and not a harmless supplement.[137] Therefore, you should always consult a doctor before use. It is by no means a standard treatment for insomnia.[138] There are specific sleep problems in which melatonin might help, but this should always be guided by a health professional. I will discuss this further in Chapter 10.

What about specific food and drinks? A recent systematic review describes that drinking milk can have a modest positive effect on objective and subjective sleep. However, often few participants are included in studies of milk and sleep.[139] According to the researchers, drinking fermented milk at night also has a positive, but small, effect. When we look at the impact of bananas on sleep, there is one fishy study that found a decrease in sleep problems in the banana-eating group, but on a vague scale for which no further reference is given.[140] In another study, subjective sleep quality improved after subjects ate two kiwis an hour before going to bed, and they slept longer.[141] However, the research setup was flawed and the fruit company Zespri sponsored the study: so perhaps take the kiwis with a large grain of salt? Elsewhere, according to a very small study, sour cherry juice was found to have positive effects on sleep: the 8 adults who consumed this beverage slept longer and had better subjective sleep quality.[142]

The type of food you eat does not only seem to influence sleep but also has an impact on how energetic you feel in the morning. The composition of your breakfast, and specifically how many carbohydrates it contains, can have an effect. One study showed that if you eat more carbs after waking up, you feel energetic faster. The researchers mention that it is important to include foods with a low GI (glycaemic index), such as low-fat dairy and a large number of fruits.[143]

Taken together, knowledge about nutrition and our night's rest is still in its infancy, which is quite strange, because more research could potentially be valuable for both producers and consumers. Methodological problems often arise in the published studies, such as few participants, little experimental research, the lack of a control group and possible unmeasured variables that influence both cause and effect. As a result, it is often not possible to make reliable statements about a causal relationship between nutrition and sleep. There are clear indications that a protein-rich diet – that would include foods such as fish, meat, nuts and seeds, and many dairy products – could help achieve a better night's rest. It is unclear what the optimal ratio between fats and carbohydrates should be due to varying scientific results.

In general, it seems wise not to eat an hour before you go to bed, but if you do, avoid eating too much fatty food. There is still the most evidence for a positive effect of milk on sleep, but unfortunately, the measured effects are small in most cases. A reason why products such as warm milk could help may also have to do with the fact that it helps to support an evening ritual. If you have learned as a child to associate warm milk with good slumber, then this alone could have a positive effect. There is some evidence for a positive effect of nutritional supplements on our night's rest: vitamin D and certain amino acids such as tryptophan could provide support, but it is always advisable to consult with a doctor when you want to use a nutritional supplement, as some supplements can have side effects, contraindications, and can even negatively affect sleep.

A diet that has received a lot of attention in recent years is intermittent fasting. With this type of diet, you limit the number of hours in the day in which you eat. For example, a schedule could be that you are only allowed to eat for 10 hours a day. Some diets are even stricter, in which you only eat for 4 hours a day. It wouldn't do for me: I get hangry just thinking about it. Research into intermittent fasting has been contradictory.[144] One study found that participants on an intermittent-fasting diet lie awake longer during the night, while another showed no difference. The risk of developing insomnia was not shown to be affected by following an intermittent fasting diet. However, researchers indicated that the studies were actually too small to draw clear conclusions.

Food is not the only thing we take that might impact our sleep. Stimulants such as caffeine and alcohol might also have an influence. In Chapter 7, I will discuss the effects of stimulants and recreational drugs on sleep. First, I am going to zoom in on social factors that influence our night's rest.

6.

Social Sleep

'One can never hate someone who has seen him sleep'[1]

Elias Canetti, *Aufzeichnungen* (1942–94)

In the prehistoric era, people slumbered together, sometimes around a campfire, which probably had a very important effect on feeling safe from dangers in the night. As mentioned earlier, in modern hunter-gatherers, couples co-sleep with their children in the same home. During the rainy season, the Hadza sleep in huts (built exclusively by the women) and during the dry season they sleep under a light covering. In a group of 33 people, 30 shared a sleeping surface with at least one other person. For married adults with children, the total number of co-sleepers could range up to 7 people, with an average of between 3–4 people sleeping together. [2]

A 2018 study of the Hadza by Alyssa Crittenden and colleagues showed that the higher the number of co-sleepers, the greater the fragmentation of sleep. Breastfeeding mothers experienced more night-time awakenings, but they still slept the same number of hours as other tribe members.[3] For men, it is common to get married around the age of 21 and for women around the age of 17. Tribe members are free to choose a partner. Sometimes a fight arises when several men want to marry the same woman; this occasionally ends violently. Monogamy is most common, but marriages are often brief. Only 20 per cent of tribe members stay with a partner for life. Tribe members are therefore usually 'serially monogamous'.

The Hadza live in camps of about 25 people, but there are often changes in the composition of such a group, with people moving in and out. Every 2 months or so, the camps are moved to another location.[4]

From this data it becomes clear that the sleep environment of a Hadza member is often busier than the average Western bedroom. They also have a different way of looking at marriage because it is normal to be married several times. Of course, this is now also the case for many people in industrialised society. You could possibly compare the change of marriage partner with the different relationships we have during our lifetime, but usually we do not move in with most partners or have children with them very quickly. What effect does a romantic partner have on your night's rest? Is it better to sleep alone or with a partner or pet in the bed? What effect do loneliness, friendships and work satisfaction have on your sleep? But also the other way around: does a good slumber affect the quality of your romantic, social and occupational functioning? I will try to answer these questions.

Romantic relationships

We do not know how people in prehistoric times fell in love, but the experience of physical attractiveness must have played an important role, just as it does nowadays. A well-rested and healthy-looking partner must have been more attractive because he or she might possibly lead to better offspring, and give better protection and care. That is where sleep comes into play. What does science say about falling in love and sleep?

When people fall in love, this can have an effect on their subjective sleep quality, though the evidence is contradictory. Two studies found a link between falling in love and dozing off more easily in adolescents. They also showed fewer awakenings and experienced fewer sleep problems during the night when they had more feelings of being in love.[5,6] On the other hand, one study indicated that female adolescents had shorter sleep times when falling in love and most studies showed no relationship between romantic feelings and sleep.[7,8] An important difference between the studies was that the ones showing a positive effect measured the subjective intensity of the feelings, while the other studies only looked at the presence or absence of these feelings.

What is the reason for a possible link between experiencing more butterflies in your stomach and a better night's rest? One of the mechanisms might be that better sleepers have a better mood and more energy, and in this way, good sleep possibly enhances the expression of sexual feelings.

Another positive aspect of good subjective sleep quality is that it can improve perceived physical attractiveness. In one study, 40 observers rated pictures of 10 individuals who either slept as usual or followed a protocol of sleep deprivation. Sleep-deprived people had more hanging eyelids, as well as redder and swollen eyes. They also had darker circles under the eyes, more pallid skin, more wrinkles and more droopy corners of the mouth. An important aspect of the study was that people were deprived of sleep for 31 hours, after which a sleep of 5 hours followed – a more extreme form of sleep deprivation than people usually experience in real life.[9] But it seems that a good night's rest can help you become a Casanova or a seductress. In a period of falling in love, where physical attractiveness and having more energy are important in the selection of a partner, the presence of good subjective sleep quality might enhance attractiveness and sexual drive. Conversely, if you sleep poorly, you probably have less desire to look for a partner and less desire for sex.

After a period of courtship, a long-term relationship may follow. What effect does your relationship have on your night's rest? There is contradictory evidence about the role of relationship status on sleep.

One study showed that there is a link between being unmarried and a poor night's rest, while another study indicated that single people sleep better.[10,11] A significant factor is that the first study included white-collar workers, while the second one examined male military personnel during the COVID-19 lockdowns. The military personnel were used to being away from home for a long time and were now unexpectedly back at home because of the pandemic. This might explain more sleep problems in the married group, who suddenly had to adapt to family life, which could be stressful.

Having a romantic partner does not always lead to a better night's rest. Science shows that the effect of a relationship depends on the quality of the bond. For example, people experienced better quality sleep when they were more satisfied with their romantic love.[12] A more positive experience of your bond also relates to sleep over longer periods. People perceiving social support from their romantic partners showed better subjective sleep quality over a period of 15 years.[13] It might be that a good romantic connection is protective for your slumber. This is logical, because less daily stress leads to a better night's rest, and some relationships can be very stressful.

Sleeping worse might also contribute to more problems in a relationship. It seems to play a role in partner conflict, and vice versa. In Chapter 3, I discussed how your night's rest can have an influence on emotions, energy levels, concentration and memory. When you are feeling tired because of sleep problems you might be less inclined to consider the other person's perspective. Indeed, poorer sleep can lead to problems being empathic and can lead to a worse mood. Conflicts are often not resolved as well as they should be when both partners sleep well. If either partner has a bad night, conflict conversations can become worse and conflicts are less easily resolved.[14] It is often said that you should never go to sleep on an argument, that you should sort out conflicts before you go to bed, and there is indeed research that supports this approach. Due to specific brain activity, negative memories can be suppressed less effectively during sleep, which can cause them to become even more prevalent. We therefore forget negative events less well. The brain structures involved in this are the amygdala, which is important for emotions, and also the hippocampus, which is very important for long-term storage of information.[15] So even if you're angry with your partner because he or she didn't do something you asked, try to get over your hurt and talk out the disagreement before going to sleep.

In extreme cases, a bad night's rest might even lead to more aggression between two loving partners. For instance, bad subjective sleep quality has a link with psychological and physical partner abuse. Specifically, research shows that a bad night's rest can exacerbate abusive behaviour.[16] You can imagine that because of this, tensions between both partners will continue to increase and that people will end up in a cycle of even worse sleep and more partner abuse.

The loss of a partner or the end of a romantic relationship often leads to worse nights. University students, for example, had more sleep difficulties after a recent breakup.[17] There is also a relationship between a high intensity of feelings of grief after the death of a partner and sleep problems. Bereaved persons in general show lower subjective sleep quality, more problems dozing off, sleeping shorter periods, and more anxiety-ridden night-time awakenings.[18]

Overall it seems that there is a strong relationship between the quality of romantic relationships and sleep. More feelings of being in love might enhance subjective sleep quality while, unsurprisingly, losing a loved one can lead to worse sleep. Probably the link between our night's rest and the romantic bond has to do with the presence or absence of stress and the feeling of happiness. In addition, positive feelings about a bond might relate to a sense of psychological safety, which also promotes a better night's rest. Aggression towards or conflict with a romantic partner is likely to have the opposite effect.

Bed buddies

Does sleeping in bed with a romantic partner have a positive effect? Studies on this topic found contradictory results. Some scientists use actigraphy to measure sleep through movement, which is less accurate than polysomnography, which measures brain activity. In actigraphy research, one study concluded that people generally slept less well when co-sleeping.[19] Another study concluded that women sleep less well when sleeping with their romantic partner and a third concluded that men sleep better when co-sleeping.[20,21]

Another study used polysomnography, which allowed the researchers to more thoroughly investigate the effects of sleeping with your spouse on your night's rest.[22] They examined 24 healthy young adults and next to subjective and objective sleep parameters, the quality of the bond was measured by using questionnaires. The study showed a greater amount of REM sleep in the couples. Interestingly, biologists found the same effect in the hyrax, a type of furry mammal which lives in groups.[23] (On a side note, the funny thing about writing about sleep and evolution is that you learn a lot of things that may be helpful when playing a knowledge board game like Trivial Pursuit or doing a pub quiz. For example, before researching this book, I was never aware of the existence of the hyrax. Now I know much more about these stumpy-toed little critters than will ever be useful.) Back to REM sleep. The researchers suggest that a more stable dream sleep might have to do with the perception of a safer environment, which allows a person to sleep better during this phase.[24]

As discussed earlier, subjective quality of sleep and quality of relationship are related, but it goes further than that. A recent study found that there is a connection between synchronisation of the brains of romantic partners during sleep and the 'depth' of their bond. To examine this, scientists measured brain activity in couples sleeping next to each other. In a questionnaire, the people had to indicate how important the partner was in their lives. The deeper the perceived connection, the more similar the partners' different sleep stages were over time.[25]

From neuroscience, we know that people's brains synchronise when they communicate with each other and that this effect is stronger in people who have a close bond.[26] This may express a physiological substrate for attachment. The fact that this even seems to happen during sleep is extremely interesting. Although the study sample was a small, homogeneous group, the first results are promising.

Though there may be a good number of positive effects of co-sleeping with your partner, in my work as a sleep therapist I saw many cases in which co-sleeping was a challenge. For example, if your partner snores, uses a CPAP machine due to obstructive sleep apnoea or tosses and turns a lot, it may sometimes be wiser to discuss whether you can sleep separately. This is still a taboo for many people, but if you consider that you function so much better after a good night's sleep, it can sometimes be an easy choice to lie in separate beds. Some people choose to sleep separately every night, while others do it every now and then. Sleeping apart is nothing to be ashamed of and is sometimes a well-considered joint choice that only shows that you care a lot about each other as partners.

Sometimes, romantic partners are not the only ones sharing our beds. As I mentioned, the Hadza sleep with an average of 2–3 bed partners: usually their children and their romantic partner. The more people in one bed, the more fragmentation of sleep, which makes sense. If you have more bed partners, it is likely your sleep will be more frequently disturbed by tossing, turning or snoring. In line with this, an Israeli study on the effect of co-sleeping on the subjective and objective sleep quality of parents and children showed that co-sleeping mothers had more fragmented sleep. Also, although these mothers reported more infant awakenings during the night, this could not be measured objectively. The researchers concluded that mothers might wake up sooner when an infant is in the bed. Another explanation is that mothers who tended to co-sleep were already worse sleepers before the baby was born, which might then make them more vulnerable to waking up because of movements or sounds of the newborn child during the night. From this, the scientists concluded that it is important to consider the quality of maternal sleep when considering co-sleeping.[27]

Next to infants or romantic partners, some people also have dogs or cats snuggled up against them during the night. Research shows that 56 per cent of pet owners sleep with their pet in the same room.[28] What effect does this have on our sleep quality? It seems that there is no negative effect of a dog sleeping in the bedroom when the dog is older than 6 months and is sleeping outside the bed. However, when the dog is in the bed during the night, the objective quality of our night's rest, as measured by actigraphy, seems to decrease.[29] In short, it is better to put Pluto in a dog basket next to the bed than have the furry little four-legged monster in the bed, where he or she can disrupt your night's rest. A funny thing is that scientists also measured sleep in the dogs who slept in their owners' bedrooms, and they showed excellent objective sleep quality!

What about the presence of a cat in the bedroom? It might be a different story than dogs. Cats are more nocturnal animals, as they tend to have their major sleep period in the afternoon. Therefore, they may be more alert when their owners are asleep. This can cause more night-time disruptions.[30] Later, I will discuss more pros and cons of our furry friends.

Taken together, having a romantic bed partner might lead to a better night's rest, in particular more stable REM sleep and a greater amount of dream sleep. The stronger the bond, the better the slumber may be. If there is a pet in your bedroom, this might not have a negative effect, as long as it is not in the bed and if it is not a cat. Sorry, Felix.

Sexual healing

Does a good night's rest promote a satisfying sex life? We know that a lack of sleep can have a negative effect. Sleep deprivation can decrease sexual desire and arousal in women and there is a link between a lack of sleep, disrupted sleep and erectile dysfunction for men.[31,32]

Not only the amount or subjective quality of sleep but also sleep timing can potentially affect sex life. For example, there is a link between shift work and erectile dysfunction.[33] However, another aspect of the night's rest might interfere with these results. One study indicated that the erectile problems mostly occurred in shift workers who also report problems in sleep quality.[34] Although there were some methodological issues in this study, it might be that subjective sleep quality problems are more important than timing when it comes to this topic.[35]

Next to subjective quality and timing, sleeping enough might also influence your sex life. As discussed earlier, short sleep can affect appearance and energy, which might have a negative effect on sexual desire. This might help explain why people who sleep worse tend to engage less in sexual activities.

Sleeping better, and enough, might promote a better sex life, but what effect does sex have on our night's rest? As I discussed in Chapter 1, the primordial cave dwellers probably did not have sex in their beds but out of sight from other tribe members. They could still benefit from the positive impact of sex on their slumber if they went to bed quickly after the deed, because research shows that it might have a positive influence on dozing off. Scientists used a survey to examine the perception of sleep and sexual activity in 780 participants. They looked at the subjective sleep-promoting effects of couple sex versus masturbation. In addition, they looked at the possible effect of an orgasm on subjective sleep quality. Orgasms with partners were sleep-promoting: reaching an orgasm after masturbation correlated with better subjective sleep quality and dozing off more easily. There were no differences between men and women in sleep improvement after reaching an orgasm in general.[36] However, after partner sex, more males *perceived* improvement in sleep quality in mixed-sex relationships than women. An explanation for this may be that in mixed-sex relationships men reach an orgasm relatively more often than women after partner sex. In same-sex relationships, women reported greater frequency of orgasm from partner sex (while there were no clear differences in same-sex relationships for men when compared to mixed-sex relationships), so it would be interesting to examine whether these women also experienced even greater subjective sleep quality.[37] Another study showed that not only having sex or reaching an orgasm might be beneficial for our night's rest; the emotional satisfaction of sexual activity was also an important factor.[38]

The conclusion is that sex with another person can be very beneficial for sleep, especially when reaching an orgasm and being emotionally satisfied with sex, and that masturbation may also have a positive effect. From research, we know that talking about sex is difficult or taboo for many.[39] However, it can probably help to discuss with your partner how you can possibly use sex or masturbation to fall asleep faster.

Why could sex have a positive effect on sleep? Relaxation might be a very important aspect. This might also explain why the degree of emotional satisfaction plays a role. Feeling more satisfied and possibly connected with your bed partner might increase feelings of psychological safety and relaxation, which makes it easier to doze off. Hormones may also play a role. When reaching an orgasm, there is a release of oxytocin in the body, as well as less production of the stress hormone cortisol.[40] Higher levels of oxytocin can lead to an overall better quality of life and a reduction of stress.[41] It seems that both the psychological and physical effects of emotionally and physically satisfying sex are very sleep promoting. So, learn to 'love' yourself a bit more if no one else does: it's healthy.

Friends with benefits

The quality of a romantic relationship might influence your night's rest, but how about social contacts, such as friends? Popularity is important to many people and a lack of friends or social contacts can cause a lot of stress. It does indeed appear to be the case that people who are better integrated into a network of friends show improved indices of wellbeing.[42]

By contrast, for the Hadza in northern Tanzania, lack of popularity does not appear to be a clear source of stress. In 2023, Piotr Fedurek and colleagues asked all tribe members who their three best friends were within their camp, and from this it could be deduced who was chosen most often. There appeared to be no difference in the cortisol levels of the more popular and less popular tribe members.[43] As mentioned before, cortisol levels can provide a reliable indication of chronic stress.[44] So it seems that less popular people in the tribe do not necessarily experience more stress. Scientists think that this has to do with the fact that the Hadza community is egalitarian. This means that there are no real status differences between tribe members.

When examining social relationships, researchers can discriminate between the number of social ties and the quality of the different bonds. This relates to the size of one's social network, but also to perceived loneliness. In one study, people who perceived that they had fewer social contacts reported more sleep problems, and a perceived worse night's rest predicted fewer social contacts. There was no link with sleep duration, only with subjective quality.[45] From this, it seems that there is a bidirectional relationship between a good night's rest and a greater number of social contacts. An explanation for this might be that people who have restless nights are often tired and have worse moods, which might lead to less social engagement. A study in which sleep-deprived people wanted more social distance than well-rested people supports this.[46]

Less social engagement, in turn, may lead to less support and more feelings of loneliness, which can contribute to feelings of stress that inhibit a good night's rest. Another study indicated that depressive feelings play a role, in which depressed people are more likely to avoid social contact and generally show more sleep problems. Loneliness seems to be a mediating factor between interpersonal stress and sleep problems.[47,48,49] Of course, the relationship between social contact and sleep is not just about how many contacts you have. If you have a lot of friends around you who demand a lot of your energy, this may even hinder your sleep. That is why, in addition to the size of your network, it is also important to look at the quality of your social contacts and the extent to which you receive support from others around you.

Indeed, when it comes to a good night's rest, one of the most important factors in the quality of social relationships is how people perceive social support. In 2018, researchers at the University of Utah found that this greater social support relates to better slumber.[50] Does social support predict better sleep or is it the other way around? Because there is a lack of bidirectional analyses, we cannot say for sure. However, there is evidence that perceived social support from family and friends can predict fewer sleep problems.[51] I can relate to that. When I am having a difficult time in my life, a chat or an arm around my shoulder from a friend or family member can take away some of the stress. And stress, as we know, is an important contributing factor for sleep problems.

It seems that social connections and sleep are interrelated. From an evolutionary point of view, bonding and establishing emotionally safe connections might have helped us survive. Social life was probably extremely important for early *Homo sapiens* in a time where sticking with the group lowered direct threat from outside.

Furry companions

Did you know that prehistoric peoples took care of dogs? Archaeologists found the Bonn-Oberkassel dog with two probable owners in a grave that dates from 14,000 years ago. Science suggests that cave dwellers may have developed emotional bonds with their canine friends.[52]

What could be a reason for the origin of the prehistoric relationship between humans and dogs? According to scientists, this may be related to primordial man sharing meat with wolves, whose domesticated descendants eventually became dogs. This is based on the fact that most archaeological sites where dog remains have been found are located in Arctic or sub-Arctic areas where humans' diet consisted mainly of meat. Man and wolf may have initially started as competitors in prey-hunting, but excess meat was probably shared with the wolves. Scientists think that this eventually led to the domestication of wolves: a mutually beneficial relationship developed whereby the incipient dogs aided humans by hunting, chasing and guarding.[53]

Next to friends and family, animals can also play a very important role in perceived support and eliminating feelings of loneliness. As I said earlier, an animal in the bed is not a good idea when it comes to sleep quality, but there are contrasting results whether owning a pet has a positive impact on your night's rest. There is more research available on dogs than on cats. According to one study, dog owners have more exercise and less difficulty dozing off.[54] From another study, we can conclude that dog owners walk an average of 3.2 km a day more than non-dog owners. In addition, they tend to sleep longer (an average of 53 minutes more per night).[55] It is not clear whether the presence of the dog itself enhances sleep duration. At most, this is an association. An important factor here is that dog owners may have more active lifestyles anyway, which could make it more likely that they choose to have a dog. At the same time, because of the active way of living, they might need more physical recovery anyway, which increases sleep duration. Another explanation might still be that a dog offers a sense of companionship, leading to fewer feelings of loneliness.

Two other studies show contrasting results. In one study, researchers did not find an association between dog ownership and sleep quality. However, on average, cat owners slept shorter.[56] Remarkably, in another study, scientists found that having a dog was associated with a greater chance of having a sleep disorder and having trouble sleeping.[57]

What could explain the difference between the studies? It seems that the age of the owner might play an important role. The studies that described a positive association between pet ownership and night's rest included participants with a mean age of around or above 65. The two studies that did not find an association or a negative association examined subjects who, on average, were much younger. It could be that the sleep-protective effects of dogs, especially, are greater for older people due to the companionship and increased physical activity (also see Chapter 5). In younger people, an opposite effect might occur because the negative effects of co-sleeping with a dog or cat might outweigh the possible positive effects on sleep in a group that is already more physically active. The study did not examine co-sleeping, but as discussed earlier, more than half of dog and cat owners sleep with the pet in their bed, and this usually has a negative effect on your night's rest. This may be due to the dog or cat moving in bed during the night, which could cause sleep disturbances.

In sum, owning a pet can be protective or it can be a burden when it comes to sleep. The direction of the effect seems to depend on the age of the owner. Older people might have more benefit because it might help alleviate feelings of loneliness and have more impact on physical activity in the case of dog ownership.

Work on your sleep

In addition to the social relationships we have in our private lives, who we work with and how we work may also influence how we sleep. While we occasionally worry about whether we can get that promotion at work and what our career prospects will look like, the Hadza seem to experience little stress about this. Research shows that hunting reputation has no influence on the stress level of tribe members. Whether you are a hunter who harvests a lot of food or not, people do not seem to sleep less because of it. The egalitarian character of the tribe might also contribute to this phenomenon.[58]

In industrialised societies, work is a more important source of stress. As we have seen, stress can disrupt our night's rest through evolutionarily based principles and work is often an important source of tension. A recent study indicated that between 1995 and 2015 general work stress increased, and that this increase was mainly due to psychological demands and higher work intensity. This in turn might have a negative influence on subjective sleep quality.[59] Sleep problems can also have an effect on how work stress is experienced.[60] In effect, most studies on this topic have found a clear negative association between occupational stress and subjective sleep quality; there is a link across various occupations, countries and regions.

In addition, several studies show that insomnia is on the rise in the working age population, with insomnia complaints increasing from 35 per cent to 38.6 per cent in over 20,000 people over a 15-year period.[61] What specific aspects of stress at work might contribute to the onset of sleep problems? In a group of more than 800 Swedish employees, a poor psychosocial work environment was associated with a more than twofold risk for onset of insomnia symptoms over a period of a year.[62] So what is a poor psychosocial work environment? According to the study, a lack of social support at work was the most important factor that could explain the effect. This is in line with the findings in social contacts, in which social support also proved to play an important role in subjective sleep quality.

Sleeplessness can also have a negative effect on industry. In 2023, Australian, Dutch and American researchers concluded that insomnia is a risk factor for workplace productivity loss.[63] This is not surprising because, as I discussed earlier, problems in subjective sleep quality can have a significant effect on mood, cognition and energy levels. Next to absenteeism, this can also lead to workplace errors and accidents. There are estimates that these problems result in annual costs of $31.1 billion in the United States alone.[64]

These findings suggest that insomnia interventions might lead to better functioning at work. Indeed, a meta-analysis in 2020 showed that cognitive behavioural therapy for insomnia (which I discuss in Chapters 8 and 9) can lead to positive results. These interventions can be effective for improving workers' subjective sleep quality and general health. In addition, they can lead to improvements in productivity, reduced burnout complaints and absence at work.[65] Increased job satisfaction might be attributed to this positive effect. One study found that insomnia not only increased feelings of hostility and fatigue, it decreased feelings of joviality and attentiveness. Sleeplessness also had an overall negative link with job satisfaction.[66]

In a nutshell, good social support at work and fewer psychological demands seem to decrease the risk of insomnia, while decreasing insomnia complaints can reduce problems at work, enhance productivity and possibly increase job satisfaction.

7.

Stimulating Sleep

'What on earth could be more luxurious than a sofa, a book,
and a cup of coffee?'[1]

Anthony Trollope, *The Warden* (1855)

Earlier I mentioned that primordial humans used stimulants such as
nicotine and psychostimulants in rituals, ceremonies and social settings. Nowadays, many people use stimulants as party drugs or for
the enhancement of direct performance. For a good night's rest, it
is important to use as little chemical stimulation as possible. What
are the effects of these substances on sleep exactly?

Coffee time

The coffee bush grows wild in parts of Africa, the cradle of man, but
there are no clear sources showing that prehistoric man used caffeine. Coffee beans were probably first eaten until they were used to
make the beverage, later in history. *Homo sapiens* is thought to have
first started consuming boiled drinks, including tea, around 1,000
BCE, so we can safely assume that cave dwellers did not wake up to a
cup of tea or coffee in the morning.[2]

Coffee, various types of tea, and energy drinks contain the substance caffeine and are nowadays widely consumed. The timing of
consumption and amount of caffeine, plus personal sensitivity and

habituation, all appear to have an impact when it comes to sleep.[3] One 2013 study indicated that 400 mg of caffeine (approximately 4 cups of filter coffee) leads to an average of 1 hour less sleep, even if you take it 6 hours before bedtime.[4] What is remarkable is that coffee can potentially have a negative effect on your sleep, but that many people do not actually experience this as such during the night. Test subjects state that they have slept well, but measuring shows that they are regularly awake for short periods. How is that possible? Good sleepers, in particular, often do not notice that they are awake for a moment because they 'forget' it, as it were. This has to do with the state of your brain and a reduced functioning of your memory when you have just woken up. Either way, according to the scientists, you should not drink caffeinated drinks after 5 p.m. A difficulty in drawing conclusions from the study is that there were few test subjects and that the 400 mg that the participants took was quite a high dose of caffeine for evening consumption.

What is the advice? How many cups of coffee can you drink and when? In 1976, Ismet Karacan and a team of researchers investigated the connection between caffeine and a night's rest. It appeared that a single cup of coffee, half an hour before going to bed, had no effect on objective sleep quality, as measured by polysomnography.[5] However, after 2 cups of coffee, taken half an hour before going to bed, sleep was shorter and more superficial. Deep sleep was also postponed somewhat. After 4 cups, these effects were even greater.

A common feature of the two caffeine studies above is that they used laboratory conditions, but a lab is not comparable to everyday practice. What about real life? In the general population, caffeine use does not appear to be associated with insomnia. Scientists examined almost 1,100 people in Iceland and Sweden. Their analyses showed that the amount of coffee people drank was not predictive of problems falling asleep.[6]

Apparently, there are clear differences in caffeine sensitivity, and most people are quite capable of adjusting caffeine consumption accordingly. Caffeine-sensitive people probably drink less coffee. In others, only more extreme use of caffeine might influence sleep. Accordingly, people consuming 8 cups of coffee (800 mg caffeine) or more per day sleep 40 minutes less on average.[7] Regular amounts of coffee consumption during the day has little effect on objective sleep quality.[8] This might have something to do with habituation. If you drink caffeine every day for a week, the sleep-disrupting effects diminish. This is the case even when it comes to higher doses in the evening.[9] If you regularly drink caffeine and want to stop, it can temporarily have a negative effect on your night's rest. It usually takes quite a while before you notice this, namely more than 27 hours after your last dose.[10]

As said, some people are physically more sensitive to the substance than others.[11] Some people can feel agitated just by taking a sip of coffee, which is probably why they drink little. This concerns about 20 per cent of the population. Age also plays a role. It turns out that you become more sensitive to caffeine as you get older.[12] If you are middle aged and take 400 milligrams of caffeine in the evening, it will generally take you longer to doze off, you will sleep shorter and the quality will be reduced. These effects are greater than among young people.

No smoke without fire

As mentioned earlier, we know that nicotine was used by ancient hunter-gatherers, but it is unclear whether parts of the tobacco plant were smoked or chewed. The first indication of tobacco smoking dates from 860 CE, long after the period of prehistoric humans. Stone pipes and pipe fragments were excavated at sites in North

America indicating use of tobacco for smoking by Native Americans at that time.[13]

In contemporary hunter-gatherer groups such as the Aka tribe there is frequent smoking of tobacco. The tobacco plant is indigenous to the Americas but was brought to Africa in the 1600s by Europeans.[14] It reached the Aka much later, around the 1800s, which means that it is not an ancient custom, when viewed from a prehistoric perspective.[15]

What is the nature of the relationship between nicotine and sleep? Are poor sleepers perhaps more likely to become addicted to nicotine, or is it the other way around? Well, nicotine does appear to have a measurable influence on your night's rest. For example, nicotine patch wearers have shorter sleep, less REM sleep and less NREM3 deep sleep than those not smoking nicotine.[16] How much nicotine you use seems to matter. In an experimental setting, smokers who used higher doses of nicotine slept worse.[17]

Although people often say that a cigarette calms them down, nicotine has a stimulating effect and can cause increased blood pressure and heart rate, which can logically lead to a negative effect on sleep.[18] Indeed, smoking is associated with reduced objective sleep quality and greater difficulty falling asleep.[19,20] The more severe the nicotine addiction, the shorter the sleep and longer the wakefulness.[21] One way to determine the severity of the addiction is to look at the time between waking up and smoking the first cigarette, the 'time to first cigarette' (TTFC). The shorter this is, the more sleep problems people experience.[22] When I first encountered this term, I immediately thought of my grandparents who always smoked very early in the morning, during their first visit to the toilet. I remember having to go to the bathroom as a child and regularly trying to hold my nose because I hated the smell of cigarette smoke.

Quitting smoking is always a good plan, but your sleep problems may temporarily increase. These effects can last up to 3 weeks.[23]

Late-night drinking

We know that alcohol was used thousands of years ago by primordial man. Contemporary hunter-gatherers, such as the Bayaka in Congo, also use it, both socially and in ritual ceremonies. Alcohol consumption among the Bayaka is high. A study of 83 tribe members showed that more than 44 per cent drank excessively: on average, a male tribe member drank 10 glasses of alcohol per week and a female tribe member 5–6 glasses.[24] By way of comparison, in the United States in 2006, average alcohol consumption per week stood at just under 4 units.[25]

People around the world often use a nightcap to help them doze off. Alcohol actually helps you fall asleep better, but as I mentioned in Chapter 1, there are also negative effects. It reduces the amount of REM sleep in the first half of the night; in the last hours, there is a lot of REM sleep and lighter and more fragmented sleep. This means that you can dream more vividly, and often remember what you dreamed better. I am not just talking about pleasant dreams, because nightmares can also occur more often after using alcohol.[26]

After a night of drinking, subjective and objective sleep quality appears to decrease significantly. Sleep studies show that, on average, your night's rest is likely to be 1 hour shorter and you will wake up more often. And as with caffeine, individuals often do not even notice that they are sleeping less well with alcohol, even though that is indeed what is happening.[27]

What does an alcohol problem do to your night's rest? Alcohol abuse and insomnia often go together. About 35–70 per cent of heavy users suffer from insomnia.[28] This group often sleeps later, less deeply and wakes up more often. And the relationship between alcohol abuse and poor sleep generally? A recent twin study found that excessive drinking is associated with insomnia at all stages of life, and that heavy drinking is more likely to predict poor sleep than the other way around.[29]

So, quitting drinking pays off when it comes to your night's rest. If you want to stop drinking excessively, the beginning can be difficult. During the first 3–5 days, you sleep more superficially and wake up more often. However, there is also good news. Sleep often improves again within 1–2 weeks. You doze off faster and sleep better and longer.[30]

Joint sleep

The earliest evidence of the use of cannabis for its psychoactive effects dates back to around 700 BCE. It concerns the remains of a European-looking man – a shaman no less – excavated near Turpan, China, alongside items that included a large cache of cannabis. How do we know this person used cannabis as a psychoactive agent? It could be that the fibres were used to make nets or clothing, which was not unusual at the time. Well, the cannabis was analysed by an international team of researchers and found to contain, among other substances, tetrahydrocannabinol, the psychoactive component of cannabis.[31]

The Aka have used cannabis for nearly two centuries. When they gather, tribe members often share a pipe or cigarette filled with cannabis with everyone in the group. Next to social purposes, they also use the cannabis because they perceive that it increases their performance: for example, they say that it can increase courage during hunting and help with ritual dance.[32]

Cannabis use carries risks. It can cause dizziness and confusion, among other things, and can be addictive. Especially when used from puberty onwards, it can increase the risk of psychosis.[33] Stopping cannabis can lead to nausea, headaches, anxiety, low mood, but also insomnia.[34] Data on cannabis and sleep can be difficult to interpret because dosages and strengths of the different kinds of cannabis can vary widely. In addition, people use it in a number of ways, with different effects.[35] Cannabidiol (CBD) and delta-9-tetrahydrocannabinol (THC) are components of cannabis that have different effects. THC mainly causes a better mood and increased sensory experience. This substance is also more likely to cause known side effects such as anxiety and dizziness. Few negative effects are associated with CBD, and it is said to have a relaxing effect.[36] On the whole, cannabis has an effect on sleep structure, depending on how much is consumed; for example, it can help you doze off faster, but it can also have the opposite effect if you take a little more.

Cannabis seems to have a variable effect on deep sleep. According to one study, you would sleep more deeply after use; according to another, you would sleep more superficially. However, it is agreed that the THC component reduces REM dream sleep.[37] There may be some positive effects of THC, however. It might improve your night's rest more than CBD. Cannabis seems to work best on sleep in people with chronic pain complaints.[38] This concerns subjective improvements and experience, because objective sleep data does not confirm that cannabis would help in any form. The positive effect could therefore be a placebo effect.[39] The risk of placebo is high here because many studies are of poor quality.

In conclusion, the effect of cannabis on sleep seems to depend on the dosage, but also on the kind of use. There are positive and negative effects on the night's rest and a better sleep experience seems to occur, especially in people with chronic pain complaints, although objective sleep research does not support this.

Upper sleep

We've seen there are clear indications that prehistoric man used uppers, or psychostimulants. The alkaloids they obtained from plants could provide a euphoric feeling and lead to hallucinations. These experiences could probably bring them into better contact with each other and with nature, and this is probably why the substances were used during ritual ceremonies.

Nowadays, in industrialised countries, psychostimulants are mainly used as recreational drugs. In addition to all kinds of health risks associated with the use of stimulant recreational drugs, there are clear negative effects on the night's rest. Cocaine increases alertness: users more often have sleep problems. The drug makes you stay awake longer, sleep shorter and have less REM sleep.[40] Long-term cocaine use is associated with shallow slumber and, conversely, an increase in dream sleep. In a 2016 study, almost no deep NREM3 sleep was measured in older, regular users. People who were cocaine-dependent only reached the deep sleep phase for 1 per cent of their night's sleep.[41] That is quite shocking, because deep sleep is so important for your day-to-day health.

About two-thirds of cocaine users also regularly use cannabis.[42] If both drugs are used, this is associated with shorter sleep. But a possible causal relationship is not clear. Short sleepers may be more likely to use cannabis because, despite the conflicting data, their experience is that it helps them to sleep better.[43]

Amphetamine (speed) and methamphetamine (crystal meth), though different substances, both seem to have many similarities in terms of their effects on a night's rest. Both have a stimulating effect which negatively affects sleep quality. Crystal meth is used much less than speed and has a far more adverse effect on the night's rest: for instance, approximately 33 per cent of chronic speed users were found to be poor sleepers compared to 95 per cent of crystal meth users.[44,45] In 1964 scientists found that amphetamine shortens REM sleep and that it takes longer for users to doze off.[46] However, there have been few more recent studies on the impact of amphetamine on sleep.

What effect does ecstasy/MDMA (3,4-Methylenedioxymethamphetamine) have? After use, it leads to restless sleep during the first

2 days.[47] There are no known studies in which the direct effect of MDMA on sleep structure has been measured. However, in 1992 scientists examined people who had used MDE, which is a substance that has similar effects as MDMA. After the participants took MDE, researchers identified an increase in wakefulness and a complete suppression of REM sleep.[48] Interestingly, people with post-traumatic stress disorder might benefit from using MDMA in therapeutic settings. This group often experiences many sleeping problems, such as insomnia and nightmares. In combination with psychotherapy, MDMA improves subjective sleep quality. These effects are still present a year after treatment.[49] Please note: this relates to expertly supervised use and not self-experimentation.

If someone stops taking uppers, what will happen to their night's rest? Stopping long-term cocaine use often temporarily aggravates sleep problems and increases REM sleep. You also see the latter when people stop taking amphetamines; they experience more intense dream experiences and, after a while, subjective sleep quality improves again.[50] Anyone quitting crystal meth will likely experience poorer subjective sleep quality, especially in the first 3 to 5 days. Dozing off takes longer, they sleep shorter and lie awake more at night. More than half of the quitters were still sleeping poorly after 5 weeks, but better than before. The other half slept reasonably to well after 5 weeks.[51]

Taken together

So, what conclusions can we draw overall about the effect of psychoactive substances on subjective and objective sleep quality?

Frequently used substances, such as caffeine, nicotine and alcohol, have a negative effect on sleep quality. There is a clear difference between sporadic, chronic and problematic use. It is also important to look at the dosage. Surprisingly, for example, as we have seen, a single cup of coffee even half an hour before going to bed usually seems to have little effect on objective sleep quality. Furthermore, most people seem to be able to dose their coffee consumption themselves, based on their caffeine sensitivity. Stopping nicotine and alcohol during or after chronic use often causes temporary poor night's rest, but leads to better sleep in the long term.

Cannabis appears to have varying effects on sleep, depending on the dosage and use of components (CBD or THC), and might have a positive effect on subjective sleep in people with chronic pain complaints.

Taking stimulants such as MDMA, cocaine and amphetamine/speed and methamphetamine usually has a negative effect on objective and subjective sleep quality. Methamphetamine seems to cause the biggest problems, but cocaine and amphetamine also create problems, in terms of ease of getting to sleep. MDMA seems to cause restless sleep, especially in the first few days after use. Abuse of cocaine and amphetamine shortens REM sleep, and discontinuation of these drugs leads to a temporary increase in REM sleep and poor objective sleep quality. After a few weeks, sleep often improves again. Chronic abuse of methamphetamine/crystal meth has the greatest long-term negative effects on sleep.

While in the days of primordial man, psychostimulants were probably mainly used on ceremonial occasions, nowadays some such substances are used as party drugs or to relax. In the next chapter, I will discuss different and possibly healthier ways to achieve relaxation.

8.

Relax!

'We cannot sleep peacefully, once we open our eyes'[1]

Pierre Reverdy, *Plupart du temps* (1945)

Our bodies enter into alert mode when we experience stress, and this alertness can hamper sleep and lead to less restful wake. Stress is a signal for the body to focus on defeating direct threat. When we are confronted with imminent danger, it is not useful to sleep a lot, because we can then react less quickly. This is why the body can actively suppress sleep when we are stressed out.

To experience less stress before going to bed, it is important to wind down your day properly. Start the winding down about 1½ hours before going to bed. Quiet, low-stress activities prepare your brain for the sleep that is to come.

Some of today's hunter-gatherers do the same. For example, they sit and chat by the fire in the evening, while the weather cools and night falls. The Ju/'hoansi (!Kung) Bushmen live in northeast Namibia and northwest Botswana. Anthropologist Polly Wiessner has examined their habits and conversations. In the late afternoon, families would come together for an evening meal, after which many would gather around fires to make music, dance or talk. While daytime conversations were mostly about topics such as foraging plans and hunting tactics, the evenings were dominated by storytelling. Over 80 per cent of Ju/'hoansi 'firelight talk' concerned symbolic stories from which lessons could be learned. Interpersonal conflicts, she noted, were often not directly expressed as they were during day-time conversations, but rather in this story form, which seemed to relieve tension. Musing and reflecting, the tribe members filled their heads less with practical concerns before going to bed. As Wiessner puts it: 'They let the issues of the day fade with the embers.'[2]

In this way, the Ju/'hoansi seem to lay a much better foundation for restful nights than people in industrialised societies do. Due to the advent of the internet and social media, our practical information absorption often continues until our last hours awake.

So, given these contemporary temptations, how can we calm our brains? After discussing the scientific background of sleep and the circumstances surrounding our night's sleep in the previous chapters, in this chapter I will give a number of practical tips and exercises for working on one of the most important pillars of sleep: relaxation.

Breathe in, breathe out

Breathing exercises can improve the night's rest.[3] Here is an exercise that can be practised during the day or evening.

- Sit in an easy chair with a straight back and make sure your feet are flat on the floor.
- Place both hands on your belly and feel how your belly goes up and down as you breathe in and out. Breathe in through your nose and out through your mouth. Feel the warmth of your hands on your belly and lower the breath down toward that spot.
- Focus your attention on each breath in and out. Do not try to force a rhythm but follow your own pattern. You may notice that your breathing becomes calmer and deeper.

Try to practise this for 5 minutes a day, sitting in an easy chair, as in the instructions above, before you do it in bed. Through this relaxation exercise, you can train your body to relax better, which positively affects your sleep.

Less on your mind

If you feel stressed when awake during the night, it is good to examine your negative thoughts. You create the illusion of danger for your brain when you ruminate a lot. Our bodies then go into alert mode. It is therefore important to figure out why you are ruminating and to address those thoughts properly. How do you do that? Maybe you have tried not to fret in bed and found that it is quite difficult. Maybe you have counted sheep in the dark, done arithmetic in your head, or tried other things to distract yourself, and still you did not manage to quiet your head. Busy or negative thoughts in bed can be predators of our sleep. How can we get rid of them?

I told you earlier about my personal experience with insomnia. The cause of my problem was mainly the busy thoughts that raced through my head. I was so busy preparing for the dance performance that I became too mentally active. The music and thoughts of the dance, the movements and rhythms that began so beautifully, became a curse because they made me feel restless in bed.

It is important to examine what circumstances might be causing you to be overactive or tense. Had I known at the time that being overactive had so many consequences for my sleep problem, I would have made better arrangements with myself and created defined times when I could be engaged in performance.

My main insight from that time is that it is not only the negative thoughts that can cause stress during the night, but also the positive ones. Engaging in many pleasurable or creative activities can lead to a poor night's rest, especially if you do not slow yourself down sufficiently in time. If you subsequently sleep worse, your thoughts may become increasingly negative.

If you want to have a better night's rest, it is a good idea to examine what conditions may be making you too active. Arrange times when you let yourself deal with the problems or challenges, but also seek adequate relaxation and distraction. Slowing down can feel like a defeat. However, by accepting your own limits, you create space and give your brain the idea of a safer environment that will help you create more rest in the night.

Even during the writing of this book, I noticed my predators lurking. Although I enjoy the process, I find that my mind can still be in writing mode when I'm lying in bed. I think of studies I could cite or anecdotes I could share. What helps me is that these days I have a far better understanding of how sleep works, which allows me to limit the times when I am working on books, and that works well. What also helps me is that I realise that my enthusiasm and drive can sometimes lead to shorter and more fragmented sleep and less restful wake. It helps when I see that, at such moments, I have a choice to be busy with many things and that the downside is that I simply sleep (and wake) differently. By seeing this more as a choice and less as something that happens to me, I create peace in my mind.

In life there are, of course, a number of situations in which you do not immediately have a choice to remove a stressful situation. For example, the death of a loved one or experiencing a traumatic event can have a major impact on your sleep over a long period of time. In my patients I saw that it can sometimes help to see being awake as part of the grief or trauma, and as part of the coping process. Resisting, rather than accepting, your insomnia at such times can often only lead to more broken nights. In other cases, I've found that patients often think that they're powerless to reduce the effects of stressful situations in their lives. But through sleep therapy they find they have more control over the situation than they'd previously thought.

Use your imagination

Primal man probably slept more shallowly when there were possible night-time dangers. In Chapter 3, we saw how an unsafe environment is associated with spending more time awake and being more restless. In modern-day life, thoughts of negative or exciting situations can create the illusion of danger; and our brains often react identically when we think about a certain situation to if we are actually in that situation. Sometimes this works to our disadvantage. For example, one study found that just thinking about fearful situations, or creating the mental imagery, leads to increased anxiety.[4] Therefore, to promote sleep, it is important to give your brain the idea that your environment is safe enough for sleep.

One method that can help you do this is visualisation. By visualising yourself in a safe place, your brain gets the signal that it does not have to check the environment and therefore it needs to be less alert. According to a 2018 study, thinking about nature-based environments can be especially effective for reducing feelings of anxiety.[5] This is not surprising because it has been shown that experiences in nature can contribute to feelings of wellbeing and stress reduction.[6] The 2018 participants were asked to imagine either being in a nature-based environment or an urban environment. The researchers found that although both imagined environments helped reduce anxiety, the reduction in anxiety from the guided nature imagery was significant.[7]

So, a caveman-style safe place check is very effective at decreasing anxiety. Here is an example of such a visualisation exercise:

- Imagine yourself in a pleasant, safe place. This could be in a forest or on a beach, or a specific safe place you remember from your childhood.
- Close your eyes and imagine what that place looks like. Imagine the colours; try to perceive what the ambient temperature is like and what sounds you hear.
- Try to focus on every detail you see, smell, hear or feel, so that you really feel like you are in that safe place.
- It is okay to take a few minutes.

The more often you practise this, the better your body will be at responding as if you were actually in that safe place. You will then become increasingly calm.

It is good to go through this exercise a few times during the day at first. You can then try doing it just before you go to sleep. Imagine lying down in that place and always remember that you are completely safe there.

When I look at my own safe place, it is a beach on a bay, near Portimão in Portugal, where I am relaxing with the sun on my face. I hear the rolling of the sea and smell a combined scent of sea air and sunscreen. I am lying on a towel and my hand touches the warm sand. When I think back about it, I actually want to go there again!

Be mindful

Various scientists have studied the effect of mindfulness-based techniques. Mindfulness stems from Buddhist traditions and refers to a state of conscious in which people show a non-judgemental awareness of experiences in the present moment, instead of trying to alter the current experience or to eliminate it from their awareness. For example: when people are confronted with negative thoughts or situations, their tendency might be to 'not think about it' or leave the situation. Being mindful means you learn to observe the thoughts or situation without judgement. Mindful methods used to enhance sleep vary from meditation – focusing on the regulation of attention and emotion, and an increase in body awareness – to therapies in which more insight is gained into metacognitive processes (learning to think about how you think about your own thoughts) to reduce emotional stress, such as mindfulness-based cognitive therapy (MBCT), or acceptance and commitment therapy (ACT).

A review of 6 randomised control trials showed that mindfulness meditation can modestly reduce insomnia symptoms. This is reflected in less time awake at night and higher subjective sleep quality.[8] Unfortunately, the number of subjects in each of the 6 studies was limited. In the review, which included both meditation and MBCT, subjective sleep quality improved after mindfulness-based stress reduction and mindfulness-based cognitive therapy for insomnia.[9] It is noteworthy that some of these treatments included psychoeducation around sleep, which often leads to better knowledge about the basic principles (such as sleep pressure and the biological clock) – which in itself can have a positive effect on insomnia complaints.

I will now describe a mindfulness exercise that can support sleep.

Have you ever tried not to think about something? Just try closing your eyes and not thinking about a pink giraffe for a minute. You will find that this is not easy! The harder you try to suppress a thought, the more it seems to force itself on you. This can be very annoying, especially when you are just about to go to sleep. What makes it extra difficult is that in bed you have little distraction from other stimuli. As a result, the thought can only get bigger and bigger.

If negative or exciting thoughts keep recurring, it may help to do a visualisation exercise that is slightly different from the previous one. The goal of this exercise is not to get rid of your thoughts, because we know that does not work. The goal is to have a different attitude toward these thoughts and create a little more distance, which might create more inner peace. Try the following:

- Imagine you are in a forest, in a clearing. You hear the rustling of leaves by the wind, and it is cold, but you feel the cosy warmth of a campfire. You may decide whether you lie there alone or have someone, or several people, with whom you feel comfortable and safe, with you.
- Again, try to imagine that place as best you can. You lie there safely, and the place is familiar. Maybe you smell the fire and hear the crackling of the wood. The fire keeps any predators at bay. Hold this environment in your mind for a moment. You may find that your mind wanders to another situation, but that is okay. Try to go back to that spot in the woods each time.
- Now imagine that you see one or more animals around where you are lying down. They are all at a safe distance because of the fire. Each animal you see represents a thought. A positive thought turns into an animal you feel good about. A negative thought turns into an animal you do not feel so good about, or maybe even a dangerous animal. It does not matter if there is a tiger or a lion, because you are safe by the fire.
- Examine the animal and all of its characteristics. How does it look, what does any fur look like and what sound does it make? Thoughts follow each other repeatedly, and so you visualise a new animal that fits your thought. If you have the same thought for an extended period, the animal stays until you have a new thought. It does not matter how long the animals are present and what sounds or movements they

make. The fire will keep them at bay, and you have time to look at them closely.

Through this exercise, you learn to allow thoughts in and to look at them with more distance. Thoughts are stories and images that our brain creates. When you do this exercise, these concoctions will have less effect on you. Thinking about events can have the same effect on you as experiencing the events themselves. Handling those thoughts differently can have a positive effect on your sense of calm and, therefore, on your night's rest.

Although relaxation might already help you get better shut-eye, there is an even more powerful way of creating a better night's rest. I will discuss this method in the next chapter.

9.

Working with Hours

'Sleeping is no small art: it is necessary to keep
awake for it all day long'[1]

Friedrich Nietzsche, *Thus Spoke Zarathustra* (1885)

In the past few chapters, I have discussed a number of factors that can help improve your sleep and create more restful nights, even when you are awake. I've talked about adjusting expectations around sleep, creating the right sleeping conditions, and reducing stress. But there's more. It is fascinating to see that a sleep pattern that we would quickly describe as abnormal or bad is very common among contemporary hunter-gatherers.

As I wrote in Chapter 5, the Hadza have an average total bed time of just over 9 hours and sleep an average of 6 hours and 15 minutes. They are awake for an average of 17 minutes before falling asleep, but during the night they are awake for almost 2½ hours. That means that the time spent in bed actually asleep – their *sleep efficiency* – was about 69 per cent. This is in stark contrast to the 85 per cent that we perceive as being sufficient in industrialised countries. Interestingly, the 85 per cent first seems to have appeared in 1989 in an article about the development of the Pittsburgh Sleep Quality Index, a general questionnaire for measuring the quality of your sleep, though there was no clear research supporting that cut-off score.[2] Despite this, clinicians and scientists used the score for decades as the gold standard for distinguishing between good and poor sleepers.

Only in 2019 did researchers find that a sleep efficiency of 83 per cent creates a better distinction between good and poor sleep.[3] The same study found that sleep times of between 5 hours 20 minutes and just over 7 hours were typical for good sleepers, which is much shorter than the general recommendation of between 7 and 8 hours for adults, given by the National Sleep Foundation in 2015.[4] In fact, the shorter sleep times from the study are very similar to the short sleep times of the Hadza. Interesting . . .

It is important to mention that both the sleep times of the Hadza and that of the 2019 study are based on actigraphy, which mainly measures movement. Research shows that actigraphy and subjective sleep duration do not always correspond; people who sleep poorly tend to underestimate their sleep duration, while good sleepers tend to overestimate their sleep duration. In one study, 34 per cent of participants showed a difference of more than an hour between actigraphy and their own estimation of sleep time; and on average, the participants thought they slept 23 minutes longer than the actigraphy indicated.[5]

What does this mean? Well, research shows that actigraphy corresponds more closely to the actual sleep duration measured during reliable polysomnography (the gold standard sleep measurement) than subjective sleep does.[6] Therefore, if you are a good sleeper and think you have slept 6 hours, you may have slept a little less. If you are a poor sleeper and think you have slept 6 hours, you may have slept more, which might be yet another relief to people with insomnia. This probably has to do with the phenomenon I mentioned in Chapter 2, in which people who have highly fragmented sleep, such as in insomnia, might subjectively experience much less rest at night. In people with insomnia, their brain only seems to register sleep after a period of over 30 minutes of undisturbed slumber. Nevertheless, in insomnia therapy we work with subjective sleep duration and subjective sleep efficiency especially, because that ultimately says something about the perceived sleep quality, which is one of the most important indices of improvement in therapy.

There is one peculiarity which has to do with the fact that the Hadza tribe members who were studied, despite having an average sleep efficiency of less than 70 per cent, do not report a sleeping problem. As we have seen, one of the reasons is probably not so much that we in industrialised societies sleep worse, but that we experience our waking hours far more negatively. As a sleep therapist, the patients I saw experienced the nights as difficult and often worried about not sleeping. You can imagine that this creates more stress and fatigue than if you are woken up a couple of times by one of your five bedmates and then lie in the bed relaxed, after which you fall asleep again.

I therefore think that insomnia is not so much a sleep problem but rather a wake problem. If you are able to lie relaxed in bed, you are less likely to experience a sleep problem. When analysing broken nights the question should not so much be: 'Why are you not sleeping' but: 'Why are you awake' and, moreover: 'How are you awake?'

It seems that the pressure on sleep and the creation of an almost unnatural super night's rest is plaguing industrialised countries. A reflection of this can be seen in the huge run on sleep medication in recent years, which has probably only taken us further away from natural sleep, which I will go further into in this chapter. After that, I will discuss the most powerful method to decrease wake time and create more rest in the night.

The magic pill?

In ancient Egypt healers mainly treated insomnia with remedies such as opium and saffron.[7] As we saw earlier, in the Middle Ages waking up at night was seen as normal, so people did not pay much attention to it.

By the sixteenth century, physicians were treating insomnia problems with ointments, pills and potions.[8] Beginning in the 1960s, doctors regularly prescribed sleeping pills in the form of benzodiazepines.

In recent years there has been a lot of support for not prescribing sleep medication or prescribing it less. There are obvious reasons for this. For example, did you know that after taking a sleeping pill, you objectively barely sleep longer, and your objective sleep quality deteriorates? This is important to know because objective sleep quality is the most important thing for your physical health and overall functioning. Research shows that 15 days after you stop taking sleep medication you objectively sleep as long again as you did while using.[9] Just after stopping, you will sleep worse for a while, because your body has become accustomed to the medication, but after that, you end up sleeping the same amount of time without medication. Moreover, your amount of deep sleep and your objective sleep quality increase considerably after stopping sleeping pills. Another drawback in benzodiazepines and nonbenzodiazepines is that they often cause reduced functioning in thinking. Both short-term and long-term use lead to problems in attention and working memory and memory for events.[10] Additionally, one study in older adults (over the age of 55) found that a specific nonbenzodiazepine drug, zolpidem, has been found to cause an increase in cognitive problems that can last up to 6 months after quitting.[11]

Nevertheless, benzodiazepine and nonbenzodiazepine use is still high in industrialised countries. Benzodiazepines are not only used to sleep better but also to reduce anxiety or relax muscles, for example. They are also the most commonly prescribed psychiatric medications.[12] More than 1 in 20 people in the United States receives a benzodiazepine prescription.[13] When benzodiazepines are used for sleep problems, the general rule is that they are prescribed for a short period (less than 4 weeks) due to the negative sleep effects, side effects and risk of addiction.[14] However, a 2018 study shows that more than a quarter of a million people in the UK are likely to take benzodiazepines and nonbenzodiazepines beyond the recommended time scales.[15] A European study shows that in insomnia patients, benzodiazepines are prescribed for an average of more than 15 weeks. There is a clear difference between the countries. In England the average is just over 7 weeks and in Germany around 11 weeks, while in Spain the average is 23 weeks.

Patients often dread the discontinuing of sleep medication, which I also call *anti-wake medication*. Their ultimate fearful scenario is that they lie stressed out in bed again with subsequent exhausting days. From my experience as a sleep therapist, I think that in most cases, the problem in quitting medication is not so much that patients want to sleep longer, but that they don't want to be confronted with their difficult experiences of restless wake again, and this, despite all the negative consequences, is exactly what the medication takes care of. People are often not aware of more natural ways of achieving more night-time rest.

To summarise: the problem with quitting sleep medication is that patients often experience withdrawal symptoms, such as restlessness, cognitive issues and temporarily worse sleep. This often causes people to continue using the medication, even though it is no longer effective and can cause negative health effects. However, in most cases it is advisable to stop, but do so only in consultation with your doctor. There are alternatives available that work long-term and can promote sleep in a more natural way. I will now discuss one of the most powerful techniques.

The alternative

The gold standard treatment and the most effective non-drug intervention for sleep problems is cognitive behavioural therapy for insomnia (CBT-i).[16] A meta-analysis shows that the treatment is effective in 70 to 80 per cent of the cases analysed.[17]

In my own study, working with colleagues at the sleep medicine centre, 60 people were treated with CBT-i and the results were impressive.[18] Most of these patients had been referred to us by their GP for insomnia treatment, and had had consultations with other sleep doctors or neurologists beforehand to rule out possible medical causes.

We first examined whether there might also be a mental health condition in addition to the insomnia. The patients were given questionnaires to measure the severity of their insomnia; variables such as personality and quality of life were included. The patients then followed a programme lasting 4–6 weeks, in which they were provided with psychoeducation about sleep: they kept sleep diaries and they received relaxation training and behavioural treatment, including sleep restriction (using shorter total bed times to sleep better) and stimulus control (getting out of bed when not able to sleep), which I will explain more extensively later in this chapter. In some cases, we also performed cognitive therapy. This addressed negative thoughts around sleep and encouraged the patients to view sleeplessness more positively, so as to lead to more relaxation and better sleep.

At the end of the treatment and in a follow-up after 3 months, we examined the extent to which they had improved in terms of sleep and whether the CBT-i treatment had had an effect. About 83 per cent of the people with insomnia without additional mental health issues reported no more symptoms at the end of treatment. They reported an average of 1 hour 20 minutes longer sleep than before treatment and reported being awake in bed only 20 per cent of the time instead of 44 per cent of the time. Furthermore, on average, they no longer needed 80 minutes to doze off, but experienced sleep onset after 24 minutes. You might expect people who have had sleep problems for some time to respond less well to CBT-i, but that was not the case.

The treatment was less effective in patients who had mental health issues in addition to insomnia. Only 23 per cent of these had no insomnia symptoms at all by the end of therapy.[19] Nevertheless, they experienced other improvements after treatment. The average time they needed to doze off decreased from about 90 minutes to 45 minutes, and they experienced an average of almost an hour longer sleep per night. Furthermore, they showed significantly fewer depressive symptoms after CBT-i.[20]

Thus, the general advice is to address both sleep problems and mental health issues if both are present.

Earlier, I discussed the role of menopause in insomnia. CBT-I is also the gold standard treatment for sleep problems during and after menopause. A 2016 study found that after CBT-i, perimenopausal and postmenopausal women indicated that they had better subjective sleep quality, fell asleep faster and spent less time awake.[21]

Not everyone has access to CBT-i treatment however, and many will need a referral to a sleep therapist, who often have long waiting lists. The good news is that sleep restriction also has great results in postmenopausal women: in a study of 150 women with insomnia, sleep restriction was almost as effective as full CBT-i.[22]

Know your sleep

The first step in learning to sleep better and be more relaxed throughout the night is to know what sleep is and how it works. After reading the previous chapters, you should be something of a sleep expert yourself, so we're already most of the way there. I will now go through the next step of the treatment with you, which is about expectations around sleep and keeping track of your own sleep through a sleep diary.

How does your knowledge of sleep contribute to a better night's sleep? It protects you from some of the 'predators' of the night. For example, it is reassuring to know that waking up briefly a few times a night is normal and that we really don't need to sleep for 8 consecutive hours to have a good night's rest. It is important to know that waking up briefly every now and then is perfectly normal. You can think of waking up in between as a little evolutionary safety check to see whether there are possible predators.

Remember that insomnia is often not so much about a lack of sleep but rather about the way you lie awake. If you attach a lot of negative value to these times, it can create stress. For example, a brief moment of waking up can degenerate into a fear that this moment will stretch for hours. Moreover, if you know that you do not necessarily need 8 hours, you will wake up feeling different after 6 or 7 hours of sleep than if you believe you had an insufficient night's rest. A change of mindset reduces stress and reduces fretting about sleep. This leads to a better night's rest. In this way, hopefully you will have chased away one predator already!

To work on your sleep, it is important to know *how* you sleep. A sleep diary can help you do that by keeping track of what your sleep looks like and if there are any changes in your sleep pattern. The diary serves as a reminder, because it can be very difficult to remember how you slept several days ago. By keeping your sleep diary, you can monitor whether your sleep improves by doing certain things differently. This gives you a better grip on your night's rest. It is also nice to visualise your progress in a diary.

If you want to improve your sleep, it is important to keep the diary for a few weeks. You will find an example of such a diary at the end of this book (see Appendix). The chart there shows you how often you were awake and approximately how long you stayed awake. You fill it in based on your feelings. Try not to fill it in very precisely and do not put it next to your bed, otherwise you will focus even more on your sleep problems, which can be stressful. Just put your diary somewhere else in the house and fill it in once you are up in the morning. Then put it back where it was. As I mentioned earlier, it is very important not to use a clock or mobile phone to check the time overnight, because this can often worsen your sleep problems.

The diary is used as the basis for one of the most effective methods – if not the most powerful method of improving your night's rest: *sleep restriction* – or lying in bed for shorter periods of time.[23] In practice, I sometimes saw patients who found it difficult to keep a sleep diary because they focused so much on sleep duration. In that case, I discussed an alternative with them, in which they only had to write down their total time in bed and perceived sleep time in the form of a numeral. Sometimes that brought a little more relaxation around sleep tracking. Some patients tended to look at their smart watches every day to determine sleep duration and quality. In many cases this is not wise when you are suffering from insomnia. I will discuss this further in Chapter 11.

Shorter might be better

It may feel counterintuitive to lie in bed for a shorter amount of time when you are experiencing sleep problems, but as we saw in Chapter 2, increasing sleep pressure can cause you to doze off faster and sleep deeper.

If you suffer from insomnia, your tendency is often to lie in bed for longer, but that is counterproductive. It can create more problems falling asleep and more fragmented sleep due to lower sleep pressure. As we've seen in the Hadza, fragmented sleep does not have to be a problem. It becomes one when you notice that it makes you restless and tense.

If we think about the evolutionary basis of our sleep, the purpose of sleep restriction is not to sleep longer or to sleep more continuously, but to make the nights more restful. By using the biological mechanism of sleep pressure, you shorten the moments in which you can worry, which ensures that you are more rested during the day. This echoes what I saw in practice. After sleep restriction therapy, people may still have been awake sometimes, but they weren't worried about it anymore. They regained confidence that sleep would come or not. Through the apparently contradictory therapy of keeping shorter total bed times, they learned to deal with sleep, and especially wakefulness, differently. For this reason, I also regularly saw people who did not sleep much longer than at the beginning of the treatment, but who still indicated that they were satisfied with their new sleeping pattern.

Sleep restriction is ultimately what helped me with my insomnia. I began to look at sleep differently within a few weeks. I slept my usual 6½ hours after 2 weeks of treatment but had more relaxed nights and felt much better during the day.

It appears that sleep restriction alone is just as effective as the full cognitive behavioural therapy treatment I described above (psychoeducation, relaxation training, stimulus control, sleep restriction and cognitive therapy). A meta-analysis in 2021 indicated that applying sleep restriction greatly reduces the severity of insomnia and that people fall asleep much faster and spend much less time awake in bed and concluded that the benefits are comparable to full cognitive behavioural therapy.[24]

Previously, only theoretical models were available that could explain the rapid and strong effects of sleep restriction. But in January 2022, it was discovered that the increase in sleep pressure and reduced arousal can actually be measured physiologically during sleep restriction.[25] An advantage of the restriction therapy is that it is widely applicable. In addition to positive results in young to middle-aged adults, there are strong positive effects in older people and the very young. Children aged 6–14 years dozed off better when their sleep pressure increased. Four weeks after treatment, parents indicated that children still fell asleep better and slept better. Significantly, no negative effects were found on the cognitive functioning of the children due to shorter total bed times.[26] In older adults (mean age around 65), sleep restriction also has clear benefits, causing them to fall asleep faster and sleep better.[27]

Then the question arises: why do few people know about this highly effective method? I have a number of hypotheses about this that I base on my clinical impressions and years of working with people with insomnia.

There is a hyperfocus on sleep duration in our society. This is based on 'old folk wisdom' – such as 'you should sleep for 8 hours' – and is sometimes reinforced by the emphasis placed in the media on 'getting enough sleep'. Even studies linking sleep quality to negative health effects sometimes translate into headlines such as 'Too little sleep leads to . . .' This gives a negative connotation to staying in bed for a shorter period. If getting enough sleep were so important, why would you reduce your chances of getting enough night's rest? The answer is simple: you have to improve subjective sleep quality first before focusing on increasing time asleep. To achieve this, staying in bed for a shorter period is often necessary. This seems paradoxical if you have always assumed that the period of time you sleep is so important.

People often think that medicating the problem is the answer. This can cause patients and medical professionals alike to overlook other approaches. Some take prescribed sleep medication, but others prefer over-the-counter pills, herbal extracts and other 'passive' treatment methods. Sleep restriction requires a change in behaviour and is therefore not as popular as the 'quick fixes' that do not work, only work a little, or even prove counterproductive in the end, such as sleep medication. Sleep restriction might be difficult in the first few days. In this period, people often report that they are sleepy and function less well. It often takes at least 1 or 2 weeks before you feel better, which scares some people off.

In addition, the term 'sleep restriction' is not very attractive. It seems as if you are limiting your night's rest and people who sleep poorly can logically drop out. 'Prescription total bed time' is a more positive term that may also be easier to use in practice.

Another form of behavioural treatment that is a very effective treatment for insomnia is stimulus control.[28] With this form of treatment, you only go to bed when you are sleepy, and if you wake up in the night, you get out of bed after 20 minutes to do something that relaxes you. When you are sleepy again, you go back to bed. With this method, you actually also apply a form of sleep restriction because you shorten the time in bed by getting out when you are awake.

Previously, it was thought that stimulus control would cause us to make less of a connection between the bed and lying awake. According to the theory, insomnia involves conditioning, whereby a person with insomnia learns to lie awake because . . . they frequently lie awake. By getting out of bed you could break this learned relationship.[29] However, a 2023 meta-analysis shows evidence that this is not the working mechanism of the method. Instead, the researchers concluded that the positive effect of stimulus control is probably more related to a reduction in cognitive activation due to distraction after getting out of bed, which breaks the negative cycle of thoughts and additional tension.[30] This also fits perfectly with the picture of today's hunter-gatherers: they don't need to get out of bed because they don't worry about waking up at night.

The positive effects of sleep restriction and stimulus control are both strong. How do you know which method to choose? In practice, I often chose to implement sleep restriction first. The reason for this was that I noticed that stimulus checks often led to even more anxiety at night. Patients told me that when they woke up in between, they were excessively concerned with whether the 20 minutes had already passed and whether it was time to get out of bed. And getting out of bed at night often felt like a punishment. The advantage of sleep restriction is that it is clear when you go to bed and what time you get up, and that you do not have to worry about what happens in the meantime. This can give many people peace of mind. I often added that the patient could get out of bed if the tension became too high at night and return when they were sleepy (again). If the patient was just lying quietly in bed, I advised them to just stay in bed, just as contemporary hunter-gatherers do.

Getting stronger

Can you perform sleep restriction on your own? Yes! In most cases, this is very effective and safe. However, in people who have epilepsy or severe psychiatric disorders, it is important to consult with your GP or health practitioner before starting the method.

Here are the steps:

- First, keep a sleep diary for a week. After that week, review how long you have slept and how long you have spent in bed, on average.
- Divide the average time you have slept by the average time you have spent in bed and multiply that number by 100. This gives you a percentage. We call this the *sleep efficiency.* Imagine you've slept an average of 6 hours and spent 8 hours in bed:

(6/8) x 100% = 75%
Your sleep efficiency is: 75 per cent.

- When you are suffering from insomnia, a sleep efficiency score below 83 per cent is considered low and might indicate that you are not experiencing restful nights. Remember that treating sleeplessness does not involve sleeping longer or staying awake for less time per se, but staying awake for less time can help you have a more restful night. That is why we work with the sleep efficiency score because it indicates how long you lie awake (including times you are feeling tense). In addition, people who do not experience insomnia may function well with a lower sleep efficiency score because they are simply more restful in bed when they are awake, just like the Hadza.
- When you experience insomnia, you increase the sleep efficiency by lying in bed for a shorter time. You determine the time you are going to spend in bed by looking at your average sleep time for the first week.
- The second week you are going to spend as much time in bed each night as you slept on average during the first week, plus half an hour. So, for example, you're going to spend a maximum of 6½ hours in bed each night. You go to bed at the same time and set the alarm clock. No matter how much or how little you slept that night, you then get up.

For many people this might sound like a challenge. Most of my clients were even more tired after the first week than before starting restriction and suffered from more concentration problems and a new complaint: sleepiness. This is quite normal. Your body has to get used to the new structure. If you are sleepier, it is a good sign. This is a consequence of your sleep pressure increasing.

During restriction, you might have all kinds of negative thoughts and want to give up, but hang in there! You can compare it to following a diet, starting a new exercise regime, or stopping drinking alcohol. Even if it is difficult, it is important not to give up during that difficult initial period but to really persevere for a few weeks. It then becomes easier to persevere.

The accumulated sleep restriction of the past few days is going to have a positive effect on your night's rest. You will notice that falling asleep and sleeping will be slightly better after a few days, which will lead to more restful nights. Despite that better sleep, you may still feel tired during the day. It often takes a few weeks before your body is completely accustomed to the new rhythm, and that means you have to persevere for a while.

The next steps are:

- You continue to keep your diary during the weeks you apply restriction and calculate your sleep efficiency weekly.
- When you score 83–85 per cent or higher for a week, gradually expand your total bed times again by 15 minutes per week.

Over time, you will find that you have found an optimal balance between your total bed time and sleep time. If your sleep efficiency score remains at least 83 per cent, that is fine! You may sleep the same number of hours or a bit longer than before sleep restriction, but your nights will be more relaxed, and that is what matters!

In line with the sleep pattern of the hunter-gatherers, you may even choose to let go of the sleep restriction a bit more at a certain stage. You can choose to do so, as long as you can accept the moments when you lie awake at night, and deal with them in a relaxed manner. However, it remains important for your circadian rhythm to maintain constant (longer) total bed times as much as possible.

Insomnia is the most prevalent sleep issue in modern society, but it is not the only sleep problem. Sleep disorders such as obstructive sleep apnoea and narcolepsy affect millions of people throughout the world. In the next chapter, I will focus on two specific sleep disorders – delayed sleep phase syndrome and parasomnia – and explain behavioural techniques which can help reduce symptoms.

10.

Clashing Clocks and Nightly Ghosts

'It was morning according to the clock, but the deepest
night in his body'[1]

Jeffrey Eugenides, *The Marriage Plot* (2011)

'We dream in our waking moments and walk in our sleep'[2]

Nathaniel Hawthorne, *The Scarlet Letter* (1850)

Cave dwellers slept in more dangerous conditions than we do now-adays, so for survival it was important that people had different biological clocks. This would ensure that at least someone was awake who could keep watch during the night.

An extreme example of this is delayed sleep phase syndrome, or DSPS. This is a sleep disorder in which a person falls asleep much too late and wakes up much too late, leading to difficulties in work and other day-to-day activities.

Another example of a phenomenon we now classify as a sleep disorder but might have been useful to prehistoric man is *parasomnia*. This is a collective term for unusual behaviour and psychological events occurring during sleep. These 'events' (another word for the occurrence of unwanted behaviors or sensations during sleep) take place as the brain transitions in and out of sleep.[3] People suffering from parasomnia might experience recurrent episodes of sleepwalking, nightmares or sleep paralysis. Such events can be frightening, and when they occur frequently, the disturbed night's rest can result in fatigue, sleepiness and problems in daily functioning.

The *threat hypothesis* gives an evolutionary explanation for these phenomena. It states that parasomnia is probably a simulation of threat which occurs during sleep.[4] This recurrent simulation leads to more practice with dangerous situations in a safe mode (sleep). It prepares you for when that threat actually occurs, day or night. In other words, if you dream about bears or sabre-toothed tigers at night, but also about a more contemporary 'threat', such as an angry colleague or being stuck in an elevator, you can respond better to it during the day. Most of us probably will not dream about predators anymore, but we will dream about things that do not work out, or difficult situations, and this can seem just as threatening to us.

In this chapter, I will discuss these two sleep disorders – DSPS and parasomnia – that we think originated a long time ago and were likely adaptive then, but which have now probably lost most of their value.

Sleeping the day away

As I stated in Chapter 2, the biological clock plays an important role in your day–night rhythm. In most cases, the rhythm of that clock sufficiently matches your desired rhythm. This means that you can perform your normal daily tasks well because you sleep at the desired time and are alert at the desired time. However, in some people, there is a clear mismatch between the biological clock and the rhythm of society, and this causes problems.

Imagine that you invariably doze off at 3 a.m. and do not wake up until 11 a.m. In that case, your biological clock has a delay, as in DSPS. The opposite can also be true. Some people are sleepy very early and wake up very early. We call this advanced sleep phase syndrome

(ASPS). Travelling through time zones can also induce a circadian rhythm problem: the jet-lag syndrome that I discussed in Chapter 2.

As a sleep therapist, I saw more patients with a delay in the biological clock than with ASPS. The reason is that people with ASPS are generally better able to meet their obligations of work or school. That said, ASPS can have strong negative consequences on your relationships and social life and can lead to loneliness. Dozing off at 8 p.m. every evening is no fun. Especially if you still want to go to that nice get-together or party.

I regularly saw clients with a delay in the biological clock who did not know what was causing this. They were changing employers repeatedly for years due to systematic tardiness. I also saw adolescents who encountered a school attendance officer because of school absenteeism. The parents of these adolescents were often at their wits' end.

Because people with DSPS are often late for work or school, or sleepy during the day, they can appear unmotivated. Consequently, those around them often react negatively to that behaviour. This, in turn, can cause individuals to feel worse about themselves, leading to withdrawal. Being away from work or school makes it even more difficult to stick to your desired rhythm. This is how you end up in a vicious circle.

Delayed sleep phase syndrome is fairly common.[5] It usually starts in puberty, when there is a natural delay in the biological clock, and children who already fall asleep late doze off even later. A complicating factor is the early start of the school day. The prevalence of DSPS decreases with age, the biological clock steadying after young adulthood. About 1 in 20 adolescents has DSPS. In contrast, the prevalence of DSPS in adults is about 1 in 600. The difficulty is that, due to their shift in the biological clock, teenagers cannot go to bed earlier to get enough sleep. They simply lie awake longer. Adolescents with DSPS can sometimes learn to cope with their sleep problem by making choices that fit their biological clock. Later in life they might find work in security, nursing at night, or in the hospitality industry – jobs that suit a late circadian rhythm just fine.

What are the causes of DSPS? One of the factors is how long the biological clock takes to complete a day. With DSPS, the clock appears to tick for an average of 25 hours before it starts again, which is half an hour longer than average. That causes you to have more trouble getting sleepy in the evening.[6] Another factor has to do with individual differences in the suprachiasmatic nucleus (the main area of the brain that regulates our circadian rhythm) in its sensitivity to light.[7] As a result there is faster inhibition of melatonin production, which hampers the night's rest. In addition, a genetic component might explain the occurrence of DSPS.[8] If your parents are late sleepers, there is a good chance that you yourself also doze off late.

Reset

DSPS can be treated by chronotherapy, combined with light therapy.[9] Chronotherapy literally means *time therapy* and involves shifting your biological clock. Light therapy involves the use of a daylight lamp. Such a lamp must produce at least 10,000 lux, which is comparable to full daylight. The light resets your internal biological clock in the morning and makes you wake up and become active faster. When shifting your rhythm, it is important to take gradual steps. In this way, bit by bit, your body adjusts to its changing rhythm.

How does chronotherapy work exactly?

- Imagine you have to get up at 7 a.m. in the morning because of work. You would like to be asleep by 11 p.m., but you repeatedly fail to doze off before 12.30 a.m. As a result, you often do not wake up until 8.30 a.m.

- The advice is to follow your natural biological clock for 2–3 days. In this example, you go to bed at 12.30 a.m. and get up at 8.30 a.m.
- After getting up, you immediately use the daylight lamp for 20–30 minutes. In the summer, you can also sit in a sunny spot in front of a window or outside.
- After 2–3 days, you go to bed half an hour earlier and set the alarm for 8.00 a.m.
- When you get up you use the daylight lamp again in the same way.
- You do this again for 2–3 days and continue like this until you arrive at your desired rhythm.

You can try this method at home if the difference between your actual time of falling asleep and your desired time of falling asleep is not more than 1½ hours. If the difference is bigger, you should consult your doctor or a qualified sleep expert.

In some cases, melatonin can support a positive shift in the biological clock. As I stated in Chapter 5, incorrect use of this supplement can cause even more sleep problems. Taking melatonin at the wrong time can have the opposite effect on your sleep. So do not experiment on your own if you have DSPS symptoms. If you decide to start taking melatonin, it is important to make an appointment with your doctor or with a qualified sleep therapist, so they can advise you on any contraindications, dosage and timing of intake.

If you have ASPS symptoms and have trouble staying awake in the evening, it may also help to use a daylight lamp, such as in the afternoon or early evening. Be careful with this lamp, however, because if you use it too late, you may actually develop sleep problems.

Next to DSPS, jet lag is a very prevalent problem in people, especially when they are travelling east. As I discussed in Chapter 2, it can lead to problems initiating sleep and create fatigue and sleepiness during the day. It can take days before the body adjusts to the new rhythm, and then you return home and the process of adjustment starts all over.

Several treatment options can help combat the problems of adjusting to a new time zone.[10] As with DSPS, an important factor here is the use of light. Seeking bright light exposure in the evening after a westbound journey and using bright light in the morning after an eastbound journey can help support the transition.[11] In some cases, taking melatonin can help in this process, especially when travelling east. However, again, it is important to consult with a physician for advice on suitability and dosage. Sometimes caffeine can reduce jet-lag-induced daytime sleepiness and increase alertness, which might help you get through the day.[12]

Mind your step!

People experiencing parasomnia often feel sleepy during the day. This is because nocturnal restlessness repeatedly disturbs the sleep. It also results in irritability, mood swings and impaired thinking. People who sleepwalk or often have nightmares may find it difficult to sleep in different places, because they are afraid of embarrassing themselves or worry that others will think of them as 'strange'. Nevertheless, it is important to inform others about such sleep problems, as colleagues or friends are more likely to understand if someone is not feeling well, falls asleep unintentionally or has concentration problems.

In some, the unusual behaviours during sleep take such extreme forms that they run outside and get into their car or even commit serious crimes. The latter is thankfully rare. The first description of a murder possibly related to parasomnia dates back to 1878. A 28-year-old man, with a history of 'night terrors', killed his infant son. The man claimed he was still asleep and thought that his son was a wild animal come to attack his family. The court did not find the man guilty, because the trial judge stated that the defendant was unaware of his act in that moment due to his somnambulism.[13] Fortunately, most forms of parasomnia do not manifest so violently.

Parasomnia can occur in different stages of sleep. In non-REM parasomnia, the behaviours and sensations occur mainly during NREM3 (deep sleep) but can also occur in NREM2 (the second stage of light sleep).[14] Examples of non-REM parasomnias are sleepwalking and sleep anxiety. Another type is *confusional arousal.* Confusion and disorientation are the main characteristics of this phenomenon, without major accompanying behaviours or autonomic responses.[3] For example, this is the case when someone briefly awakens and looks around without knowing where they are but does not get out of bed. Sleep eating and sleep sex (*sexsomnia*) are also forms of non-REM parasomnia. People who have these sleep disorders do not usually consciously experience them and cannot recall eating or performing sexual acts.

If you are a parent, you may have noticed that your child is sometimes restless at night. For example, you suddenly hear a loud yelp or scream coming from your son or daughter's bedroom at night. When you go to look, you see that they are sitting upright in bed with eyes wide open, but you cannot seem to make contact. This is an example of another NREM sleep phenomenon, namely *nocturnal anxiety.* It is important not to wake your child in these situations, as this can only cause more distress. Usually, children go back to sleep after a few minutes, and in the morning they often do not remember what happened the night before.

Parasomnia is more common in young children than in teenagers or adults. For instance, the prevalence of confusional arousals in children between the ages 3–13 years is just over 17 per cent; above the age of 15 it drops to almost 7 per cent. Under 12 years of age, sleepwalking occurs in 17 per cent and sleep terrors in 6.5 per cent.[15]

Why is parasomnia more common in childhood? It turns out that the boundaries between sleep and wake in our brains are not yet fully developed in children.[16] This causes behaviour that you normally exhibit when you are awake to also occur during sleep. Parasomnia is also hereditary. This may explain why you are more likely to sleep-walk if your father or mother was a somnambulist.[17]

Scary dreams

Unwanted sensations can also occur during REM sleep. Two-thirds of people have had a nightmare at one time or another.[15] As I mentioned earlier in Chapter 3, dreams or nightmares often take different forms, depending on the culture and threats a person may encounter on a daily basis. This means that a hunter-gatherer may be more likely to dream about wild animals and a student may be more likely to dream about being socially excluded at college.

Maybe you recognise a dream in which something or someone chases you, but you cannot move forward. You suddenly wake up bathed in sweat and need to recover.

Nightmares take place in REM sleep. Because they often have a strong emotional value, you can often remember them well. This is a big difference with a non-REM parasomnia. Here, you often cannot remember or can remember the sleep phenomenon in much less detail. Another distinction between both types of parasomnia is that REM parasomnia occurs more often in the second half of the night. This makes sense because most REM sleep occurs during that period.

Have you ever experienced waking up in the morning and not being able to move your body? It could be that you have experienced *sleep paralysis*. At such a time, you want to move but cannot. You are not able to talk, so you cannot call for help. In addition, you may see or experience things that are not there at all. You may even have the experience that something or someone is pressing on your body so that you cannot move yourself. In the eighteenth century this phenomenon was depicted by Henry Fuseli in his painting *The Nightmare* (1781): a woman lies stretched out across a bed, her head and upper body hang over the edge, and a large demon sits crouched on her chest. Sleep paralysis occurs because there is a mismatch between our brain and body.[16] Parts of our brains are awake, but our bodies still exhibit the characteristics of REM sleep. On top of that, you cannot use your muscles.

REM sleep behaviour disorder, or RBD, is another form of REM parasomnia. Patients experiencing this sleep disorder can use their muscles during REM sleep, which can lead to unsafe situations. If you dream about a burglar in your house and you slap him in your dream, it is a good thing that you do not carry this out in real life. In RBD, patients sometimes hurt their bed partner or might get into dangerous situations because of their sleep disorder. As you can imagine, this can have negative effects on your relationship, and on how you view your sleep: after all, you are going to be far less relaxed in bed if you know that unpleasant things can happen during the night. An important distinction with non-REM sleep disorders is that people can remember what they dreamed more accurately in RBD. It can be associated with various neurologic disorders, such as multiple sclerosis and Parkinson's disease.[17,18] Therefore, it is always good to see your doctor when these specific events occur.

Triggers

Sleep deprivation can trigger parasomnia. Thus, after several short nights, you may experience an exacerbation of your symptoms. Taking certain medications and alcohol can also increase your symptoms. As with insomnia, you can also fall into a vicious circle with parasomnia. Stress can increase your symptoms. If you fret, it can worsen your sleep problem, and it can cause you to delay going to bed, which negatively affects sleep. You may start using alcohol or narcotics to unwind, which then usually backfires. The moment the symptoms increase, you start worrying more again, and so the problems worsen.

The basic principles of parasomnia treatment are largely similar to the principles of insomnia treatment.[19] An important difference is that sleep restriction is usually not a part of the treatment, because total bed times that are too short can increase the problems, especially in NREM parasomnias.

People with parasomnia often talk about feeling threatened during sleep. One example is a client who in her sleep believed that someone was throwing a stone statuette at her, causing her to dive out of the way, after which she stumbled out of bed in real life. Another client hid in his closet at night, waking up confused after having the experience that someone was chasing him. For people with parasomnia, these kinds of experiences can be very frightening. They may start fretting about it during the day, thinking they are weird or that there is something wrong with them on a psychological level. The moment they find out that parasomnia is an evolutionary relic, and that it is more common than they thought, there is often already more peace around the night. They may feel less shame and better understood.

Creating good sleeping conditions is at least as important in parasomnia as it is in insomnia.[20] In Chapter 5, I gave some advice on how to improve those conditions: the advice around bedtimes, naps, adequate light exposure during day and night, temperature, and that exercise can help reduce the problems. Some medications, such as antidepressants, antipsychotics and benzodiazepines, can elicit or aggravate parasomnias.[21] Consulting your doctor is important if you are using one or more of these medications and experience parasomnia events.

In addition, there are certain actions you can take to help yourself if you are experiencing parasomnia. Of course, it is important that you do not injure yourself while sleeping, so do not put your bed under a window to avoid unsafe situations. If you get out of bed often during sleep, it may be wise to put your mattress on the floor. When you get out of bed during sleep, parasomnia can sometimes take on extreme forms. A young man I treated for his condition had even jumped off his balcony once while sleeping. Those around him worried that it was going to happen again. By using a bell mat (a mat that activates an alarm when weight is applied) located next to his bed, he became aware of getting out of bed during his sleep. Over time, the sound of the bell was enough to make him go back to bed peacefully. If you have parasomnia, as part of your own safety, it is important to remove objects you can trip over and avoid having sharp objects in your sleep environment.

The smallest movements or noises during the night can cause an 'event' in someone with parasomnia. This is another word for the occurrence of unwanted behaviours or sensations during sleep. Environmental stimuli in the bedroom can often trigger an event. Think of everything you feel or hear during sleep. For example, if you and your partner lie together on a small mattress, you might get a parasomnia event when he or she turns over in bed. Maybe you have a partner who pulls the covers their way while sleeping. That too can lead to an event. Therefore, the best thing to do is lie on separate mattresses under separate comforters. If there is noise around you in your bedroom, it can negatively affect your night's rest. Therefore, make sure you lie in a quiet place. If your bedroom is adjacent to a busy road, it is better to try a different sleeping place. If noises during your sleep are unavoidable, use earplugs. If your bedroom is not dark enough, make sure there is adequate blackout by using blackout curtains or use a sleeping mask. The light from passing traffic or another external light source at night can also trigger events.

If you experience parasomnia, make sure you are in bed long enough. Sleeping for too short a time can actually cause more events. Also, do not lie in bed for too long: the moment your subjective sleep quality decreases due to excessive total bed time, it could cause more events. So, finding an optimum of your time in bed is important. What can help you with this is keeping a sleep diary, as described in the previous chapter. You will then get a good picture of your total bed time and sleep time and you can investigate what your optimal sleep duration is. For a few weeks, keep track of how often you experience your symptoms at night, and if necessary, adjust your total bed time a bit. If your symptoms subside, you know you are on the right track.

Worrying and negative thoughts can cause your brain to become overactive and make your body more likely to exercise at night to deal with impending danger, leading to more events. The relaxation exercises I recommend in Chapter 9 for insomnia can help with parasomnia.[22] If you experience a lot of physical or mental stress, it is important to look at your activity patterns. People with parasomnia often allow themselves little rest during the day. The agitation experienced during the day then translates to the night, which can lead to fretting, rumination or a busy head, which in turn can lead to more events.

Tame the nightmare

Sometimes, traumatic experiences or stressful events induce nightmares. Using or discontinuing medication can also lead to recurrent bad dreams. For example, the use of beta-blockers or the discontinuation of tricyclic antidepressants such as imipramine can induce nightmares, because of an imbalance in substances in the brain, so-called neurotransmitters.[23,24] Scientists explain that this can hamper the processing of emotions (as I discussed in Chapter 2) that usually occurs during a fearful dream. Instead, the negative dream is reinforced and is more likely to occur again.[25]

In non-REM parasomnia, you often cannot recall the sensations during an event or can only vaguely recall them. Usually, a partner or parent is better able to indicate whether you had one or more events during the night.

If you suffer from (recurring) nightmares, it is a good idea to write down the content of your nightmare in as much detail as possible and visualise it again during the day. So, keep a dream diary. If you regularly visualise your unpleasant dream during the day, you will find that the anxiety during the nightmare decreases more and more at night.[26] This is because you get used to the images by thinking about them during the day, with the result that they also become less stimulating.

The next step is to change your nightmare. You do this by imagining a different ending to your unpleasant dream and visualising the nightmare with that different ending. As a result, your nightmares become less frightening.[27] How does that work? I will describe an example:

- Imagine you regularly dream that you are being chased by a monster. It is a big monster with a scary, twisted face. You are running down the street and it seems like you can hardly make any progress. The monster gets closer and closer, and you feel more and more hunted and tense.
- If you have this dream regularly, you might start by visualising the nightmare in its current form every day.
- After doing that for a few weeks, try making up a different ending that fits logically within the dream. For example, you can imagine the monster falling over and not moving forward. You can now run slower until you are far enough

away from your monster. You find that you regain some peace of mind because the danger has passed.

- By writing down this new ending in detail, and then visualising it for 10 minutes every day, you begin to experience the new ending in your dreams as well. As a result, you often see the nightmare decrease in severity and frequency at night.

The final way to get a better grip on your nightmares is to learn to dream lucidly.[28] This method involves learning to recognise that you are dreaming during your nightmare. You can practise this by regularly asking yourself a number of questions during the day, such as:

'What am I doing here?'

'What was I doing 15 minutes ago?' and,

'How did I get here?'

If you do this often enough during the day, you will find that you will start doing this in your dreams as well. As a result, you are more likely to realise that you are having a nightmare and that the dream images do not match reality. This is because most dreams are not quite right. For example, one moment you are on the street and then suddenly you are in a building. Being aware of this lack of logic during your dreams causes the nightmare to lose its power. We call this lucid dreaming.

After learning about the evolutionary basis of sleep in general, why we sleep, what the effects of a bad or short sleep are, what helps maintain a good sleep, how you can reduce sleep problems around insomnia, DSPS and parasomnia, it is time to take a sneak peek into the future. What lies ahead of us in the realm of sleep?

II.

The Future of Sleep

'All our dreams can come true if we have the courage
to pursue them'[1]

Pat Williams, quoting Walt Disney in
How to Be Like Walt (2004)

The behaviours and environment of modern *Homo sapiens* have changed rapidly over the last few hundred years. This change continues and it is interesting to see what lies ahead of us in the field of sleep.

Recently, some companies have tried to simulate ancient environmental factors that might help promote sleep and circadian rhythms. Consumers are offered products such as sleep robots and handheld breathing pacers that, according to the manufacturers, should lead to more relaxation and ultimately better sleep. Other product developers have focused on reducing the effects of nightly disturbances, with noise-cancelling earplugs and white noise machines.

Let us have a look at what research on these new products shows us. Are they really helping us to sleep better, is there a placebo effect, or are they merely useless and expensive products that cater to the feelings of people who are desperate in their search for a better night's sleep? In addition, what is sleep science going to be like in the near future?

Do numbers tell the tale?

In modern times, people feel an increasing urge to get to grips with their own health via new technologies. Smartphones have functions that indicate how many steps you've taken in a day, blood pressure meters are sold in pharmacies, and smartwatches can measure your activity levels, as well as your body temperature, blood oxygen levels and heart rate. Some even claim that they can track stress levels by measuring electrical currents on the surface of the skin. Users can opt-in to end-of-day reports of dropping and spiking stress levels to help identify patterns that might explain why they are feeling stressed out. There is the idea that everything related to health should be expressible in figures and that this gives a good representation of how you are doing physically.

Many smartwatches also measure sleep quality, which translates into a 'sleep score', and fancy graphs show what percentage of REM and NREM sleep has been achieved over the last couple of nights. The questions arise: first, are these measurements accurate, and second, do they help create a better night's rest? Does it make sense to express sleep in numbers?

As I mentioned in Chapter 2, polysomnography is the gold standard for measuring objective sleep. An important characteristic of this sleep examination is, next to other factors of interest, that it measures brain activity. Devices currently available to consumers cannot measure this aspect. Most wearables use accelerometers, heat-flux sensors and optical blood flow sensors to indicate sleep or wake.[2] In addition, they try to give an impression of which phase of sleep you are in.

Several studies have compared consumer sleep technologies with polysomnography and concluded that most devices and apps are not helpful in the estimation of sleep phases, but can give a reflection of total sleep and wake time in healthy individuals who do not have insomnia.[3,4,5] A recent literature review concluded that there are new promising techniques that make wearable devices more accurate. Examples of these techniques are photoplethysmography (measuring changes in blood volume), artificial intelligence (which helps to make better computations), and new measurements such as heart rate variability.[6]

However, interpretating results is often difficult, as manufacturers regularly use vague and undefined terms, such as 'sleep score'. This can lead consumers to place value on a score that may not be well founded. As I mentioned earlier, as a therapist I frequently encountered people who only felt worse if they saw a low sleep score on their smartphone, while it was unclear what this score meant and on what it was based. A recent review study concluded that newer apps are quite reliable in measuring sleep stages in normal sleepers.[7] But how you interpret that data is key here. For example, 10 per cent deep sleep may be enough for one person to function properly, while someone else needs 20 per cent. There is also a lot of personal variation in this.

So how much stock should you put into these sleep scores? I think that in most cases it is important to just go with your gut feeling. If you are a normal sleeper and want to keep track of your rhythm and the variations you have in the amount of sleep, a consumer application may be something for you. For people with insomnia, tracking sleep using devices and apps without professional treatment is not advised, because they are not reliable enough to measure sleep duration or sleep stages. In patients with insomnia, a tracker generally overestimates total sleep time. In studies, one device performed better at estimating total sleep time but underestimated deep sleep and overestimated light sleep. Wearable devices are most suited to healthy individuals to support general wellness and lifestyle modification.[8] In patients with sleep problems, it is a concern that consumer sleep technologies might lead to a preoccupation with checking sleep – a condition known as 'orthosomnia' – and an increase of insomnia complaints.[9]

When people with insomnia are treated by a sleep professional, who can carefully interpret the results of a sleep tracker and can make sure the patient isn't constantly checking, a wearable device might aid cognitive behavioural treatment. Research shows that the advantage is not so much that the use of an app leads to better treatment results, but that it can remove the burden of keeping a sleep log.[10]

So, to sum up, sleep trackers are becoming more accurate in the estimation of sleep. In normal sleepers, they are good at measuring sleep and noting waking – new applications can even reliably estimate sleep phases. However, the interpretation of results, such as sleep scores, is not clear or reliable. Even if your sleep phases are reliably measured, it remains difficult to estimate what this means for you because there is a lot of individual variation in what is a healthy score. In people who do not have insomnia, the advice is not to use trackers to monitor sleep without professional guidance as results are less accurate in this group when it comes to sleep and wake states. In addition, unguided use can lead to an aggravation of insomnia symptoms caused by over-frequent checking. If people with insomnia are in treatment, a tracker may be able to support the monitoring of sleep, for example during cognitive behavioural therapy.

Social media influencers

People get their information about sleep from different channels and social media is a growing source of sleep information. However, the possible evidence for this information is often not checked and people can be misguided. There are many examples on social media of sleep advice which is not supported by research. An example recently circulating on TikTok and Instagram was the idea that taping your mouth shut at night should lead to better sleep quality and less snoring.

Data is available on mouth-taping and sleep, though this is mainly focused on a small sample of obstructive sleep apnoea patients.[11] Again, researchers did not examine regular sleepers but a very specific group with a very specific sleep disorder. In this study, mouth-taping led to a reduction of snoring and sleep apnoea complaints. This might in turn lead to an improvement of sleep quality in this group. The catch is that some influencers interpreted these results to mean that every sleeper would benefit from mouth-taping, while this can be dangerous without professional direction as it can lead to hampered breathing (among other things). Nevertheless, the effect was that many celebrities and athletes started promoting mouth-taping.

Is the role of social media here a bad thing? I think it is. In general, it is very important to give clear information on what type of intervention is suitable and for which group of people. Those who are experiencing insomnia might get the idea that mouth-taping is the solution for them, but this can be misleading and potentially dangerous. The same goes for influencers advocating certain types of vitamin pills and supplements to promote better sleep. As we saw in Chapter 5, the sleep-enhancing effects of most supplements are not evidence-based. It is essential that consumers make well-considered decisions when buying a product, and know if claims for its efficacy are based on scientific findings or not.

Another example of social media influencers going wild is the '5 a.m. club'. Many influencers promote people getting up very early, saying it will help their circadian rhythms and create more energy. This does not take into account that there are many people with eveningness who, if they feel the pressure to join in with this trend, might deprive themselves of (even more) sleep by getting out of bed even earlier. Again, a clear scientific basis for such statements is missing, and it might be harmful for some people to follow this advice.

The more positive side of the work of many social media influencers is that they often have large global audiences and very persuasive ways of imparting ideas. Scientists could learn from this. I think a big problem in sleep science is that many very good scientists are not able to communicate information and reach large audiences in attractive ways. Both influencers and scientists have a responsibility to spread accurate sleep knowledge and could benefit from each other's strengths: one group by backing up their statements with scientific research and the other by conveying information in ways that are more accessible and impactful. In the future, I hope they will combine forces more often. For now, always consult your doctor or sleep expert first and don't rely on the opinion of that celebrity influencer!

White noise and robots

People often use a range of products to support sleep. Think of sleeping masks, earplugs, your own pillow or duvet that you take with you on holiday, the right sleeping clothes or socks for bed, valerian drops, sleeping tea. The consumer industry cleverly responds to people's need to find different goods to help them sleep better. More and more technological gadgets are coming onto the market every day.

Will the future be full of people using robots in and around their bed to sleep better? Will they have machines that can enhance their night's rest? This may sound like a freaky idea, but the truth is that there is already a sleep robot on the market, which many people use.

The robot looks like a bean-shaped cushion and gives guidance to calm down a user's breathing by making a breathing-type motion and playing sounds or music that is intended to be relaxing.[12] The problem with many new technologies, especially start-ups, is that there is not much money to do scientific research. This often leads to a delay before scientists know whether the new product actually helps to create better sleep. Data on the sleep robot showed that in a group of 44 people, insomnia complaints did not significantly reduce and different measures of sleep, anxiety and depression did not respond to the use of the robot after 3 weeks of use. Researchers concluded that the robot was not an effective method for reducing symptoms in patients with insomnia.

The lack of positive results for the sleep robot is in line with earlier statements I made about improving sleep – the most effective way of treating insomnia is sleep restriction. It is just as effective as full cognitive behavioural treatment (CBT-i). The sleep robot intervenes in bad sleep by promoting relaxation, which might help people be more at ease before falling asleep or support them in their waking moments, but it may not be enough to remove the enormous stress that many people experience when they can't sleep. It would be interesting to examine whether people following a sleep restriction programme might benefit from the sleep robot as an add-on to the 'treatment-as-usual'.

The use of sound is another intervention that has attracted interest in the last few years. Often people refer to the continuous noise used to promote sleep as 'white noise' – noise that contains all audible frequencies in equal measure – but this is often not correct. It can be white noise, but there are other types, such as pink noise (which has fewer high frequencies) or brown noise (which has even fewer high frequencies than pink noise). The thinking is that continuous noise masks disruptive noises in the bedroom and that this promotes better sleep quality. Studies have concluded that continuous noise might help people doze off more quickly and lead to less fragmented sleep; however, the quality of the evidence is very low.[13] This mostly had to do with small groups of research participants. On the other hand, in a group of people with severe tinnitus, continuous noise did seem to reduce problems in falling asleep.[14] Another study, however, found that it might in fact disrupt sleep or induce hearing loss in healthy subjects.[15]

Another way technology is dealing with noise in the bedroom is by eliminating it as much as possible. An example of this is the use of earplugs that provide almost complete noise cancellation. You can imagine that removing noise can lead to improved sleep quality, and indeed, noise-cancelling earplugs do have a positive effect on sleep: research in healthcare shift workers shows that they experienced better sleep quality, reduced tension and less daytime sleepiness.[16] However, it is not clear to what extent electronic earplugs perform better than conventional earplugs.

In sum, research looking at the effectiveness of new technologies in improving sleep is still in its infancy. We need larger-scale studies to examine whether devices and technological aids can really help us sleep better. In the meantime the best approach is to use these products as add-ons to proven treatment strategies, such as sleep restriction, rather than using them as standalone therapies, and focus on the basic principles that help us sleep better. These I believe have more to do with the past than with the future. Knowledge about keeping balance in our bodies and mind in this rapidly changing environment is essential. For a good night's rest, it seems best to follow the natural and ancient needs of our bodies. I will discuss a wrap-up of my findings in the next and final chapter.

12.

Balance is Key

'Deep nights give us the balance of a stable life'[1]

Gaston Bachelard, *La poétique de la rêverie* (1965)

In this chapter I'll summarise the main points of this book and conclude with a 12-point plan for a better night's rest.

From research conducted with contemporary hunter-gatherers, we can deduce that primordial humans slept mainly during the night with shorter naps during the day and that there were night-time variations between tribes in sleeping in one or two periods. Being awake at night was probably a normal phenomenon and a consequence of lower sleep pressure caused by longer total bed times. In addition, nocturnal waking was a good way of coping with possible night-time threats. Next to these regular nocturnal wake periods, natural variations in eveningness and morningness probably helped to extend the period in which one part of the tribe could watch over the other tribe members, ensuring they could have a restful night and recover well from the day.

Delayed sleep phase syndrome (DSPS) is an extreme chronotype that might have helped to guarantee safety for sleeping tribe members until deep into the night. It can be hereditary, but behavioural treatment usually helps. The same goes for parasomnia. The threat simulation hypothesis gives an evolutionary explanation for the occurrence of events such as sleepwalking, sleep paralysis and nightmares. These sleep phenomena might help us deal with real threats better when we have already encountered them in our sleep. You can see this as a sort of 'virtual reality' training for coping with real-life dangers.

Biological aging of the sleep system might have also helped *Homo sapiens* throughout evolution. The sentinel hypothesis states that the increased fragmentation of night's rest in older adults might have supported survival of the human species. They were probably the ones who were more easily startled at night when there were signs of danger. The same goes for people who have high sleep reactivity and higher objectively measured REM-sleep fragmentation.

You might have been surprised to find that our ancestors probably didn't get an average of 8 hours of sleep – more like 6 or 7 hours. Based on self-reports and actigraphy, the average sleep duration of adults around the world is the same, with a lot of variation around that average. It seems that an optimal sleep duration of 8 hours in adults is an exaggeration based on outdated early nineteenth-century ideas. This 'rule' often has negative effects on those already struggling with insomnia complaints. Most people are not even able to experience that amount of uninterrupted sleep even when circumstances are optimal. Six hours of subjective sleep can be normal, as can 8 hours, though most of us fall somewhere in between.

If you are a good sleeper wondering if you sleep enough, you might try to extend your total bed time by 15–30 minutes per week and see if you function better during the day after this period. If you are a bad sleeper, it helps to focus on the quality of your night's rest first (including reducing restless wake), before looking at the hours you sleep.

The different phases of sleep all have their own characteristics. While deep sleep, or NREM3, is important for physical recovery and health, REM sleep enhances emotional memory and is important for mood and coming up with creative solutions. Light sleep

(NREM1 and NREM2) might be important for decision-making in the case of simple tasks and may improve alertness.

From an evolutionary perspective, this is a very smart design. For direct survival, it is important to have a healthy, smoothly functioning body that can respond immediately. Therefore, deep sleep is probably built in the first hours of our night's rest. It ensures that bodily processes, such as muscle growth and the boost of the immune system, still take place when you do not have a lot of time to sleep. This might especially be the case in threatening situations when predators or hostile tribes, or modern threats like money or school worries, are lurking around the corner. The repeated occurrence of light sleep and short awakenings during the night ensures a repeated possibility to check whether the environment is safe throughout the night.

Our bodies are still pretty much the same as those of our cave-dwelling forebears; evolution does not operate at the speed of environmental and technological change. When threat confronted an ancestor, it would have been logical to sleep less and watch out for danger more during the night. Our current threats are often less external and more emotional and psychological, but our brains still react in the same way. More anxiety leads to an anxious body that wants to react to threat. Thus, in this case, sleeping deeply and without interruption would not be logical. In contrast, when we relax, we put our body and brain less in a fight-or-flight mode. In our ancestors, being relaxed would have created the feeling that it would be safe to sleep well. For us, this has the same effect. Greater relaxation leads to fewer problems falling asleep, less fragmentation of sleep and more restful wake. Breathing exercises and mindfulness exercises can help achieve this. Next to this, it is important to examine the balance of activity and rest in your life. Positive stress and excitement can also create a state in the body and mind which makes it more difficult to maintain a good night's rest.

Being awake at night is normal, but it becomes problematic when the wake time is restless. It is not beneficial to stay in the bed any longer if you are tense or when you have had enough sleep. This has no evolutionary value and contradicts what happens in our bodies. Long bed times decrease levels of adenosine in the brain – a neuro-modulator involved in storing and releasing energy throughout the body – and lowers sleep pressure, which can create more fragmenta-tion of sleep and, in the case of insomnia, lead to more restless wake. While flashy headlines might suggest otherwise, our bodies are resili-ent, and periods of bad sleep probably do not have the extreme negative effect on our health as some books or media reports sug-gest. There is not much solid evidence for insomnia causing mortality or chronic disease.

As I discussed earlier, it is natural that you sleep for briefer periods and have more restless wake when you are stressed. Many people experience stress from their sleep problem or other factors, leading to a vicious circle, as was the case in my personal situation. When you experience insomnia and are in bed for too long, sleep pressure drops and you might then experience even more restless wake. In the case of stress and a relatively long length of bed times, sleep restriction is very effective. Note that sleep need will likely vary during your life and at different points you might need less sleep than you did before. The balance between total bed times and sleep need is more import-ant than holding on to a fixed number of sleep hours.

Looking at the natural environment of current hunter-gatherers, we can safely conclude that our ancestors lived in an adaptive way with environmental influences, such as light and temperature. When it was dark and the temperature dropped, they would sleep; a rise in temperature and light would give their body a boost to start their day. In the morning and afternoon, it is important to expose yourself to daylight, just as our ancestors did. In the evening, a decrease of environmental light is important. A couple of hours before bed, the amount of light should not be more than the light equalling 10 candles. While sleeping, the environment should be pitch-dark. When the night sets in, ambient temperature drops in a natural environment. To create a good night's rest, you could simulate this in the evening by turning down the heating in your living room and not making the bedroom too hot. For our ancestors it would not have been logical to go out hunting immediately before going to bed. Likewise, it is best not to exercise too intensively within 1 to 2 hours before going to bed. In general though, exercising, along with eating healthily and avoiding fatty foods, can help to support sleep.

Archaeological evidence suggests that our ancestors probably used psychostimulants in the form of alkaloids from plants during ceremonies. From this, it seems that they did not always create the perfect circumstances around sleep because they had other priorities. In general, stimulants can have a negative effect on the night's rest. However, the media often exaggerates the negative effects of caffeine, especially when you are a regular user of caffeine and are not the caffeine-sensitive subtype. Smoking, alcohol, uppers and downers all have a negative effect on sleep. In people with chronic pain, CBD might help to enhance subjective sleep quality.

The overall conclusion of this book is that during the modern age we have become far removed from knowledge about the natural processes that determine our sleep. A metaphor I often use to describe how strangely we sometimes now act around sleep is the analogy of eating a good meal. Enjoying food depends on a number of factors. First, you have to make sure the preparation of the meal is good. No one is keen on a burnt piece of meat and rock-hard potatoes. In addition, it is important that you are sufficiently hungry before starting the meal. Now imagine being very tense while sitting at a table full of delicacies. Chances are you will not be able to eat much at all. No matter how good the meal looks and how good the food smells, you are less likely to succeed in eating.

Preparing for a sumptuous meal is akin to creating good sleeping conditions: low ambient light in the evening and an ambient temperature that is not too high just before you go to bed. Hunger corresponds to sleep pressure: in both eating and sleeping, the longer you do not do it, the more your body expresses the need for it. The stress you might experience whilst you eat your meal is similar to the stress that can get in the way of a good night's rest. Imagine trying to wolf down a poorly cooked meal after eating half a bag of chips, the tension preventing you from getting a bite down your throat. That will probably not work out. If you then expect to eat anyway, it will only backfire. You might get nauseous.

So, poor sleep conditions combined with low sleep pressure and stress or tension cause a poor night's rest. Getting frustrated because you cannot get more sleep might increase the tension further. After all, expecting to sleep well in poor sleep circumstances is like expecting to consume enough of a poorly cooked meal. With little sleep pressure, trying to sleep anyway is like eating while satiated. Trying to force sleep while you are full of adrenaline is like forcing a meal down your throat.

In addition, in industrialised countries we have come to see sleep as eating in a fast-food restaurant where we are served food quickly. We are no longer used to taking a relaxed break in between courses, and we are no longer used to lying awake at night like most contemporary hunter-gatherers do. This leads to restless wake in many of us. Fast food or fast sleep is the new standard, which causes tension, especially in those who show predisposing characteristics for restless nights, such as subjectively measured high sleep reactivity or objectively measured higher REM-sleep fragmentation.

Cave dwellers most likely did not ruminate on sleep problems because being awake more at night was the standard and could actually help them survive. Therefore, they did not force longer or more continuous sleep on themselves, as we so often try to do. If you want to create good sleep, it is probably best to listen to your body and follow the natural rules of evolution. If you are a poor sleeper, try asking yourself what a primal human would have done. Do not expect to sleep uninterrupted, especially when you are very busy or when you are uncomfortable. Stress and tension are the predators of your sleep. Like me, you too may experience sleep problems without any apparent cause at the time. If this is the case, check to see if you are overactive, and if you can create more space to relax. Keep your inner predators at bay, accept your body's natural balance, and sleep and wake like a primal human would!

How to get a better night's sleep in 3 weeks

A 12-point plan

1. Don't believe everything you read or hear about sleep

Many things you think you know about sleep are probably incorrect and have to do with a distortion of reality due to problems with scientists not placing research data in their correct context, or with unscientifically substantiated cultural trends. Flashy, clickbaity, 'newsworthy' media reports can further reduce the reliability of information about sleep that reaches us. If you read messages that say nothing about how sleep is measured, what exactly is measured, or how statements about causal relationships are substantiated, ignore them. Go back and reread this book – it contains only the scientifically proven facts about sleep.

2. Let go of the 8-hour rule

It is common to sleep between 5 hours 20 minutes and just over 7 hours, as objectively measured by actigraphy. To this you should add about 23 minutes because, generally, we tend to overestimate our own sleep. This means that an average good length of subjective sleep is between just under 6 hours and almost 7½ hours. However, this varies person to person – so you need to experiment to find your personal optimum sleep length.

3. Use a sleep diary (Appendix) to record your subjective sleep pattern over 3 weeks.

This will give you an idea of how you think you are sleeping and allow you to compare it to how you feel. Don't watch the clock while you are in bed, because it might lead to more restlessness. Instead, fill the diary in every morning for 3 weeks based on your perception of sleep. For people with insomnia, it is best to avoid smartwatches or apps to measure sleep because, for this group in particular, they are less reliable. Additionally, it can lead to increased sleeplessness because people with insomnia might focus too much on improving sleep scores, which creates more tension. Measure the effect of the other 11 points of this sleep plan during these 3 weeks by using the sleep log and your daily functioning as a reference.

4. Discover your personal sleep needs

If you sleep fairly continuously but feel like you are getting too little sleep, you can extend your total bed time a bit. If you continue to have restful nights and function better during the day or even feel less sleepy, you know you're on the right track with your longer total bed times. If you are in bed a relatively long time and experience a lot of fragmented sleep while not feeling rested during the day, you might be oversleeping, in which case, shortening total bed time might help you feel more alert and rested.

5. Examine your attitude towards lying awake at night

Realise that it is normal for us to lie awake at night. We have forgotten how to lie awake because, in industrialised countries, we are faced with higher sleep pressure due to shorter total bed time. In a more natural situation, where even the best sleeper lies awake a lot (such as the Hadza), lying awake takes on a different and less problematic form. Also, make sure that you are not lying awake because of too much caffeine, nicotine or other stimulants.

6. Shorter total bed times might be better

Insomnia is more of a wake problem than a sleep problem – it is mainly not even about lying awake, but about *how* you lie awake at night. Awake time is only a problem if it's restless or anxious. If you find yourself regularly awake and restless in the night, institute a shorter total bed time to increase sleep pressure. The goal at first is not to sleep better, but to have shorter periods of restless wake. This is how you break the negative circle of insomnia.

7. Focus on the reason for lying awake rather than on the reason for not sleeping

Stress causes us to have more restless nights. This can manifest itself in lying awake more in terms of duration, but also in lying awake more restlessly. Don't ask yourself why you don't sleep, but rather examine why you lie awake so restlessly.

8. Reduce stress

To reduce daytime or nocturnal stress, use mindfulness or relaxation exercises, but also look at structural stressors in your life and remember that you often have a choice in how you allow those things to become a predator of your night.

9. Keep regular bedtimes

The basis of our sleep is a strong circadian rhythm. Strongly varying the time at which you go to bed is not supportive, so keep a regular rhythm in bedtimes.

10. Follow the rules of nature

Reconnect with nature and use natural light during the day and less (artificial) light in the evening. Create an ambient temperature drop in the evening. Even thinking about nature can help you achieve better relaxation. Use your body in a natural way by doing exercise and walking (preferably in nature).

11. Respect your personal circadian rhythm

Skip the 6 a.m. exercise class if it does not fit with your natural circadian rhythm. Try to find out what your biologically determined day–night rhythm is and try to follow it as much as possible.

12. Don't tempt the night-time ghosts

Realise that nightmares and sleepwalking probably have an evolutionary basis and that sufficient rest during the day, removing stressors at night, and keeping sufficiently long total bed times can help you reduce the symptoms.

Appendix

The sleep diary

A sleep diary is a great way to track your sleep, and this is the standard one I use in my practice. You can download a printable version from https://www.williamcollinsbooks.co.uk/wp-content/uploads/sites/43/2024/10/sleep-diary-a4.pdf

The weekly schedule runs from Day 1 to Day 7. Whole hours are indicated by a vertical bar and divided into 4 x 15-minute boxes. The bar runs from 8 p.m. in the evening to 8 p.m. the next day. It is important that you do not fill in the diary until the morning. And do not look at the alarm clock at night; fill in your best estimate.

You fill in the sleep diary as follows: Fully colour the time you spend asleep in bed, and indicate the time you were awake in bed by shading those boxes. Indicate the time you turn off the light to go to sleep with a vertical line. Each box represents 15 minutes. Round up the time you go to bed, fall asleep, wake up and are in bed, or stay in bed, to quarter-hours.

An example:

You went to bed at 10.30 p.m. At 11 p.m. you turned off the light, and you fell asleep at 11.30 p.m. You woke up at 8 a.m., but you stayed in bed for another hour and got up at 9 a.m. You went to sleep at 2 p.m. and napped for 30 minutes. The same thing happened at 5 p.m. This last time, however, the sleep lasted 10 minutes.

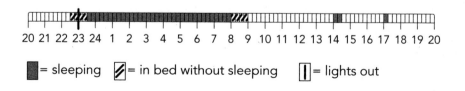

20 21 22 23 24 1 2 3 4 5 6 7 8 9 10 11 12 13 14 15 16 17 18 19 20

█ = sleeping   ▨ = in bed without sleeping |I| = lights out

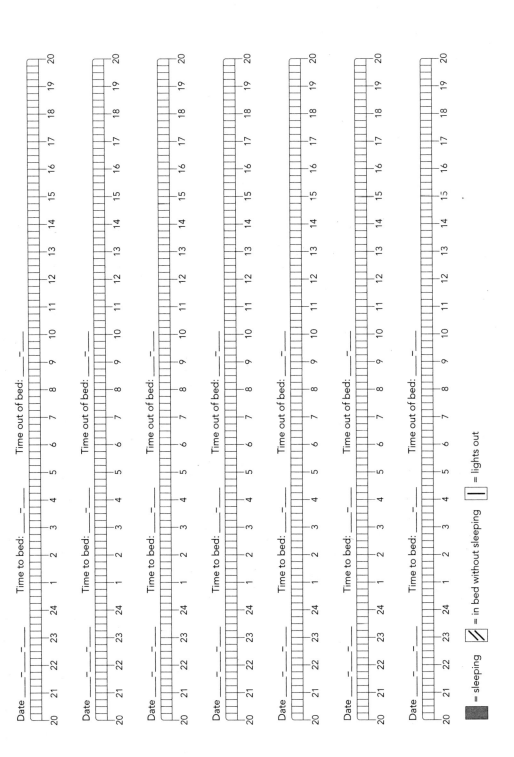

Date ___ – ___ – ___   Time to bed: ___ – ___   Time out of bed: ___ – ___

20   21   22   23   24   1   2   3   4   5   6   7   8   9   10   11   12   13   14   15   16   17   18   19   20

Date ___ – ___ – ___   Time to bed: ___ – ___   Time out of bed: ___ – ___

20   21   22   23   24   1   2   3   4   5   6   7   8   9   10   11   12   13   14   15   16   17   18   19   20

Date ___ – ___ – ___   Time to bed: ___ – ___   Time out of bed: ___ – ___

20   21   22   23   24   1   2   3   4   5   6   7   8   9   10   11   12   13   14   15   16   17   18   19   20

Date ___ – ___ – ___   Time to bed: ___ – ___   Time out of bed: ___ – ___

20   21   22   23   24   1   2   3   4   5   6   7   8   9   10   11   12   13   14   15   16   17   18   19   20

Date ___ – ___ – ___   Time to bed: ___ – ___   Time out of bed: ___ – ___

20   21   22   23   24   1   2   3   4   5   6   7   8   9   10   11   12   13   14   15   16   17   18   19   20

Date ___ – ___ – ___   Time to bed: ___ – ___   Time out of bed: ___ – ___

20   21   22   23   24   1   2   3   4   5   6   7   8   9   10   11   12   13   14   15   16   17   18   19   20

Date ___ – ___ – ___   Time to bed: ___ – ___   Time out of bed: ___ – ___

20   21   22   23   24   1   2   3   4   5   6   7   8   9   10   11   12   13   14   15   16   17   18   19   20

= sleeping   = in bed without sleeping   = lights out

Glossary

actigraphy – an objective method of measuring limb movement activity via a small recording device

adenosine – a natural substance that promotes sleepiness

alkaloid – an organic compound of plant origin which has pronounced physiological actions on humans

Alzheimer's disease – a progressive neurological condition

amygdala – a structure deep in the brain primarily associated with processing emotions

anabolic – relating to the stimulation of protein synthesis and muscle growth

bedtime – the usual time someone goes to bed

bed time – see total bed time

chronotype – A body's natural inclination to sleep at a certain time

circadian rhythm – the physical, mental and behavioural changes an organism experiences over a 24-hour cycle

cortisol – a hormone produced by the adrenal cortex that helps the body respond to stress

declarative memory – how your brain processes factual information that can be described with language, such as names, dates and facts, as opposed to skills like riding a bicycle

delayed sleep phase syndrome (DSPS) – a sleep disorder in which a person falls asleep much too late and wakes up much too late, leading to difficulties in work and other obligations

eveningness – the characteristic of being most active and alert during the evening

glycaemic index – a measure of how quickly a food can make your blood sugar rise

hippocampus – a structure in the brain that is important for long-term storage of information

hypertension – persistently raised arterial blood pressure

insomnia – habitual sleeplessness

insulin – a hormone produced in the pancreas which regulates the amount of glucose in the blood

lux (symbol: lx) – a unit of illuminance

mEDI, or melanopic equivalent daytime illuminance – a circadian metric accounting for a wide range of physiological effects of light

melanopic – describing the part of vision related to melatonin and to the circadian rhythm

melatonin – a hormone produced by the pineal gland in the brain that helps control the body's sleep–wake cycle

morningness – the characteristic of being most active and alert in the morning

narcolepsy – chronic neurological disorder that affects the brain's ability to control sleep–wake cycles

nondeclarative memory – memory accessed performatively rather than through recollection, for example riding a bicycle or running a maze

NREM (non-rapid eye movement) sleep – a state of sleep that occurs regularly during a normal period of sleep with intervening periods of REM sleep. It comprises: NREM1 (first stage of light sleep), NREM2 (second stage of light sleep) and NREM3 (deep sleep)

obstructive sleep apnoea (OSA) – a sleep disorder in which obstruction of the upper airway occurs

olfactory – relating to the sense of smell

paleo- – relating to old, ancient or prehistoric; also, another name for the Paleolithic diet

parasomnia – collective term for unusual behaviour and psychological events occurring during sleep

polysomnography – a systematic process used to collect physiologic parameters during sleep

post-traumatic stress disorder (PTSD) – a mental health condition caused by experiencing or witnessing a terrifying, very stressful or frightening event

prehistoric – relating to or denoting the period before written records

primordial – existing at the beginning of time

REM sleep – a kind of sleep that occurs at intervals during the night and is characterised by rapid eye movements and more dreaming

sentinel – a guard whose job is to keep watch

sleep deprivation – a situation or condition that occurs from a lack of sleep

sleep pressure – the need or pressure for sleep that accumulates during wakefulness

sleep reactivity – the degree to which stress exposure disrupts sleep, resulting in difficulty falling and staying asleep

suprachiasmatic nucleus (SCN) – a structure in the brain that regulates circadian rhythm

total bed time – the total time in which someone is in the bed

Acknowledgements

First, I want to thank my clients. They opened up to me about their stories and I learned a lot from them. I am glad that I was able to meet some beautiful people in my work and that they allowed me to be part of their journey to a better night's rest.

Ingrid Verbeek, you are a good friend, a fine colleague and an excellent sleep therapist. Your enthusiasm about sleep and sleep therapy made me enthusiastic and the subject will never let go of me either.

I want to thank my publishers who have shown confidence in the subject and in me. Without them, it would not have been possible to share my knowledge and experience with so many people.

Special thanks go to Sebes & Bisseling Literary Agency and to Paul Sebes for his critical view and support in the process of publishing this book.

Danny Franse, Nadine van der Laan, Yvonne van Baars, Mandy Langenhuizen, Arie de Jong and Laurens Hulshof: thank you for reading along and giving inspirational feedback. Great to have such good friends and colleagues! I want to thank my parents, Jan and Marly van de Laar, and my love Sam Mulders for supporting me in all aspects of my life – without you this book would not have been possible.

Notes

1. An Ancient Sleep

1. Dawkins, R. (1979). *The Blind Watchmaker*. W.W. Norton and Co.
2. de Castro, J.M. & Martinon-Torres, M. (2022). The origin of Homo sapiens lineage: When and where? *Quaternary International*, 634: 1–13.
3. 'What was the first PC?', Revolution: The First 200 Years of Computing. Computer History Museum: https://www.computerhistory. org/revolution/personal-computers/17/297
4. Wolf-Meyer, M. (2016). *The Hunter-Gatherers of Tanzania, Volume 3*. University of California Press.
5. Marlowe, F. *The Hadza: Hunter-Gatherers of Tanzania*. Vol. 3. Univ of California Press, 2010.
6. Kappeler, P. (1998). Nests, tree holes, and the evolution of primate life histories. *American Journal of Primatology*, 46: 7–33.
7. Coolidge, F. & Wynn, T. (2009). *The Rise of Homo Sapiens: The Evolution of Modern Thinking*. Wiley-Blackwell.
8. Wadley, L., Esteban, I., de la Peña, P. *et al.* (2020). Fire and grass-bedding construction 200 thousand years ago at Border Cave, South Africa. *Science*, 369: 863–866.
9. Hakbijl, T. (2002). The traditional, historical and prehistoric use of ashes as an insecticide, with an experimental study on the insecticidal efficacy of washed ash. *Environmental Archaeology*, 7: 13–22.
10. Wadley, L., Esteban, I., de la Peña, P. *et al.* (2020). Fire and grass-bedding construction 200 thousand years ago at Border Cave, South Africa. *Science*, 369: 863–866.

11. Walker, R.S., Hill, K.R., Flinn, M.V., *et al.* (2011). Evolutionary history of hunter-gatherer marriage practices. *PLoS ONE*, 6(4): e19066.

12. Smith, E.A. (2004). Why do good hunters have higher reproductive success? *Human Nature*, 15: 343–364.

13. Hewlett, B. & Hewlett, B.S. (2010). Sex and searching for children among Aka foragers and Ngandu farmers of Central Africa. *African Study Monographs*, 31.

14. Gray, P.B. (2013). Evolution and human sexuality. *American Journal of Physical Anthropology* 152: 94–118.

15. Konner, M. & Eaton, S.B. (2023). Hunter-gatherer diets and activity as a model for health promotion: challenges, responses, and confirmations. *Evolutionary Anthropology*, 32(4): 206–222.

16. Milton, K. (2000). Hunter-gatherer diets – a different perspective. *American Journal of Clinical Nutrition*, 71(3): 665–667.

17. Cordain, L. (2012*). The Paleo Diet Revised*. John Wiley & Sons.

18. Ungar, P.S. & Teaford, M.F. (2002). *Human Diet: Its Origin and Evolution*. Greenwood Publishing Group.

19. Jew, S., AbuMweis, S.S. & Jones, P.J. (2009). Evolution of the human diet: linking our ancestral diet to modern functional foods as a means of chronic disease prevention. *Journal of Medicinal Food*, 12(5): 925–934.

20. Larsen, C.S. (2003). Animal source foods and human health during evolution. *Journal of Nutrition*, 133(11): 3893S–3897S.

21. Zucoloto, F.S. (2011). Evolution of the human feeding behavior. *Psychology & Neuroscience*, 4: 131–141.

22. Cordain, L. (2012*). The Paleo Diet Revised*. John Wiley & Sons.

23. Zhou, J., Kim, J.E., Armstrong, C.L., *et al.* (2016). Higher-protein diets improve indexes of sleep in energy-restricted overweight and obese adults: results from two randomised controlled trials. *American Journal of Clinical Nutrition*, 103(3): 766–774.

24. Phillips, F., Chen, C.N., Crisp, A.H., *et al.* (1975). Isocaloric diet changes and electroencephalographic sleep. *The Lancet*, 2(7938): 723–725.

25. Bassett, D.R. Jr, Wyatt, H.R., Thompson, H., *et al.* (2010). Pedometer-measured physical activity and health behaviors in United States adults. *Medicine & Science in Sports & Exercise*, 42: 1819–1825.

26. Lieberman, D.E., Kistner, T.M., Richard, D., *et al.* (2021). The active grandparent hypothesis: physical activity and the evolution of extended human healthspans and lifespans. *Proceedings of the National Academy of Sciences*, 118(50): e2107621118.

27. Duke, D., Wohlgemuth, E., Adams, K.R., *et al.* (2022). Earliest evidence for human use of tobacco in the Pleistocene Americas. *Nature Human Behaviour*, 6(2): 183–192.

28. McGovern, P.E., Zhang, J., Tang, J., *et al.* (2004). Fermented beverages of pre- and proto-historic China. *Proceedings of the National Academy of Sciences*, 101(51): 17593–8.

29. Wang, J., Liu, L., Ball, T., *et al.* (2016). Revealing a 5,000-year-old beer recipe in China. *Proceedings of the National Academy of Sciences*, 113(23): 6444–8.

30. Guerra-Doce, E., Rihuete-Herrada, C., Micó R., *et al.* (2023). Direct evidence of the use of multiple drugs in Bronze Age Menorca (Western Mediterranean) from human hair analysis. *Scientific Reports*, 13(1): 4782.

31. Nunn, C., Samson, D. & Krystal, A. (2016) Shining evolutionary light on human sleep and sleep disorders. *Evolution, Medicine and Public Health*, 1: 227–43.

32. Ibid.

33. Snyder, F. (1966). Toward an evolutionary theory of dreaming. *American Journal of Psychiatry*, 123(2):121–42.

34. Yetish, G., Kaplan, H., Gurven, M., *et al.* (2015). Natural sleep and its seasonal variations in three pre-industrial societies. *Current Biology*, 25: 2862–2868.

35. Mantua, J., Gravel, N. & Spencer, R.M. (2016). Reliability of sleep measures from four personal health monitoring devices compared to research-based actigraphy and polysomnography. *Sensors (Basel, Switzerland)*, 16(5): 646.

36. Samson, D.R., Crittenden, A.N., Mabulla, I.A. *et al.* (2017). The evolution of human sleep: technological and cultural innovation associated with sleep-wake regulation among Hadza hunter-gatherers. *Journal of Human Evolution*, 113: 91–102.

37. Marlowe, F. *The Hadza: Hunter-Gatherers of Tanzania.* Vol. 3. Univ of California Press, 2010.

38. Berbesque, C.J., Wood, B.M., Crittenden, A.N., *et al.* (2016). Eat first, share later: Hadza hunter-gatherer men consume more while foraging than in central places. *Evolution and Human Behavior*, 37(4): 281e286.

39. Samson, D.R., Crittenden, A.N., Mabulla, I.A. *et al.* (2017). The evolution of human sleep: technological and cultural innovation associated with sleep-wake regulation among Hadza hunter-gatherers. *Journal of Human Evolution*, 113: 91–102.

40. Samson, D.R., Crittenden, A.N., Mabulla, I.A., *et al.* (2017). Chronotype variation drives night-time sentinel-like behaviour in hunter-gatherers. *Proceedings. Biological Sciences*, 284(1858): 20170967.

41. Ekirch, A. (2005). *At day's close: night in times past.* W. W. Norton and Co.

42. Samson D.R., Manus, M.B., Krystal, A.D., *et al.* (2017). Segmented sleep in a nonelectric, small-scale agricultural society in Madagascar. *American Journal of Human Biology*, 29(4).

43. Samson, D.R., Crittenden, A.N., Mabulla, I.A., *et al.* (2017). Hadza sleep biology: Evidence for flexible sleep-wake patterns in hunter-gatherers. *American Journal of Physical Anthropology*, 162(3): 573–582.

44. Samson D.R., Manus, M.B., Krystal, A.D., *et al.* (2017). Segmented sleep in a nonelectric, small-scale agricultural society in Madagascar. *American Journal of Human Biology*, 29(4).

45. Samson, D.R., Crittenden, A.N., Mabulla, I.A., *et al.* (2017). Hadza sleep biology: Evidence for flexible sleep-wake patterns in hunter-gatherers. *American Journal of Physical Anthropology*, 162(3): 573–582.

46. Samson, D.R. (2021). The Human Sleep Paradox: The Unexpected Sleeping Habits of *Homo sapiens*. *Annual Review of Anthropology*, 50(1): 259–274.

47. Carbonell, E., Mosquera, M., Rodríguez, X.P., *et al.* (2008). Eurasian gates: the earliest human dispersals. *Journal of Anthropological Research*, 64: 195–228.

48. Samson, D.R., Crittenden, A.N., Mabulla, I.A., *et al.* (2017). Hadza sleep biology: Evidence for flexible sleep-wake patterns in hunter-gatherers. *American Journal of Physical Anthropology*, 162(3): 573–582.

49. Yetish, G., Kaplan, H., Gurven, M., *et al.* (2015). Natural sleep and its seasonal variations in three pre-industrial societies. *Current Biology*, 25: 2862–2868.

50. Samson, D.R., Crittenden, A.N., Mabulla, I.A., *et al.* (2017). Hadza sleep biology: Evidence for flexible sleep-wake patterns in hunter-gatherers. *American Journal of Physical Anthropology*, 162(3): 573–582.

51. Quack, H. (1911). *The socialists: persons and systems. Part 2: the first thirty years of the nineteenth century.* Van Kampen and Son.

52. Yetish, G., Kaplan, H., Gurven, M., *et al.* (2015). Natural sleep and its seasonal variations in three pre-industrial societies. *Current Biology*, 25: 2862–2868.

2. What is Sleep?

1. Wertheimer, E. (1897). *Aphorisms*. Deutsche Verlags-Anstalt.

2. Webb, W.B. (1974). Sleep as an adaptive response. *Perceptual and Motor Skills*, 38: 1023–1027.

3. Siegel, J.M. (2005). Clues to the functions of mammalian sleep. *Nature*, 437(7063): 1264–1271.

4. Mora, C., Tittensor, D.P., Adl, S. *et al.* (2011). How many species are there on Earth and in the ocean? *PLoS Biology*, 9(8):e1001127.

5. Siegel, J.M. (2008). Do all animals sleep? *Trends in Neurosciences*, 31(4): 208–213.

6. Hobson, J.A. (1967). Electrographic correlates of behavior in the frog with special reference to sleep. *Electroencephalography and Clinical Neurophysiology*, 22(2): 113–121.

7. Cirelli, C. & Tononi, G. (2008). Is sleep essential? *PLoS Biology*, 6(8): e216.

8. Mukhametov, L.M. (1987). Unihemispheric slow-wave sleep in the Amazonian dolphin, *Inia geoffrensis*. *Neuroscience Letters*, 79(1–2): 128–132.

9. Koops, K., McGrew, W., Matsuzawa T. & Leslie, K.A. (2012). Terrestrial nest-building by wild chimpanzees (*Pantroglodytes*): implications for the tree-to-ground sleep transition in early hominins. *American Journal of Physical Anthropology*, 148: 351–361.

10. Nunn, C.L. & Samson, D.R. (2018). Sleep in a comparative context: investigating how human sleep differs from sleep in other primates. *American Journal of Physical Anthropology*, 166: 601–612.

11. Nunn, C., Samson, D. & Krystal, A. (2016) Shining evolutionary light on human sleep and sleep disorders. *Evolution, Medicine and Public Health*, 1: 227–43.

12. Cajochen, C., Reichert, C.F., Münch, M. *et al.* (2023). Ultradian sleep cycles: Frequency, duration, and associations with individual and environmental factors: A retrospective study. *Sleep Health*, 10(1): Supplement pp. 52–62.

13. Ibid.

14. Wielek, T., Del Giudice, R., Lang, A., *et al.* (2019). On the development of sleep states in the first weeks of life. *PLoS One*, 14(10): e0224521.

15. Sadeh, A., Mindell, J.A., Luedtke, K. & Wiegand, B. (2009). Sleep and sleep ecology in the first 3 years: a web-based study. *Journal of Sleep Research*, 18(1): 60–73.

16. Roffward, H.P., Muzio, J.N. & Dement, W.C. (1966). Ontogenetic development of the human sleep-dream cycle. *Science*, 152(3722): 604–619.

17. Jenni, O.G. & Carskadon, M.A. (2000). *Basics of Sleep Guide.* Normal human sleep at different ages: Infants to adolescents, Sleep Research Society, pp. 11–19.

18. Carskadon, M.A. (1982). The second decade. In: C. Guilleminault (ed.) *Sleeping and Waking Disorders: Indications and Techniques.* Addison-Wesley, pp. 99–125.

19. Carskadon, M. & Dement, W. (2005). Normal human sleep: An overview. In: M.H. Kryger, T. Roth & W.C. Dement (eds) *Principles and Practice of Sleep Medicine*, 4th edition. Elsevier Saunders, pp. 13–23.

20. de Mairan, J. (1729). *Observation Botanique.* Histoire de l'Académie Royale des Sciences.

21. Harding, E.C., Franks, N.P. & Wisden, W. (2020). Sleep and thermoregulation. *Current Opinion in Physiology*, 15: 7–13.

22. Mills, J. (1964). Circadian rhythms during and after three months in solitude underground. *Journal of Physiology*, 174: 217–231.

23. Yadlapalli, S., Jiang, C., Bahle, A., *et al.* (2018). Circadian clock neurons constantly monitor. *Nature*, 555: 98–102.

24. American Academy of Sleep Medicine. (2014). *The International Classification of Sleep Disorders – Third Edition (ICSD-3).* American Academy of Sleep Medicine.

25. Jagannath, A., Taylor, L., Wakaf, Z., *et al.* (2017). The genetics of circadian rhythms, sleep and health. *Human Molecular Genetics*, 26: 128–138.

26. Fischer, D., Lombardi, D., Marucci-Wellman, H. & Roenneberg, T. (2017). Chronotypes in the US - Influence of age and sex. *PLoS One*, 21: 12e0178782.

27. Randler, C. & Rahafar, A. (2017). Latitude affects Morningness-Eveningness: evidence for the environment hypothesis based on a systematic review. *Scientific Reports*, 7: 39976.

28. 'The siesta for Spanish people (La siesta entre los españoles). Simple Lógica: https://www.simplelogica.com/en/la-siesta-entre-los-espanoles-diciembre-2016/

29. Ekirch, A. (2005). *At day's close: night in times past.* W. W. Norton and Co.

30. Borde, A. (1547). *A compendious regiment, or dietary of health.* Trübner & Co.

31. Boyce, N. (2023). Have we lost sleep? A reconsideration of segmented sleep in early modern England. *Medical History*, 67(2): 91–108.

32. Descartes, R. (1632). *Treatise on man.* Reprinted 1972. Harvard University Press.

33. Reichert, C.F., Deboer, T. & Landolt, H.P. (2022). Adenosine, caffeine, and sleep-wake regulation: state of the science and perspectives. *Journal of Sleep Research*, 31(4): e13597.

34. Descartes, R. (1632). *Treatise on man.* Reprinted 1972. Harvard University Press.

35. Xin, Q., Yuan, R.K., Zitting, K.M., *et al.* (2022). Impact of chronic sleep restriction on sleep continuity, sleep structure, and neurobehavioral performance. *Sleep*, 45(7): zsac046.

36. Borbély, A.A. (1982). A two process model of sleep regulation. *Human Neurobiology*, 1(3): 195–204.

37. Deboer, T. (2018). Sleep homeostasis and the circadian clock: Do the circadian pacemaker and the sleep homeostat influence each other's functioning? *Neurobiology of Sleep and Circadian Rhythms*, 5: 68–77.

38. Maspero, C., Giannini, L., Galbiati, G., Rosso, G. & Farronato, G. (2015). Obstructive sleep apnea syndrome: a literature review. *Minerva Stomatologica*, 64(2): 97–109.

39. Buysse, D.J., Reynolds, C.F. 3rd, Monk, T.H., Berman, S.R. & Kupfer, D.J. (1989). The Pittsburgh Sleep Quality Index: a new instrument for psychiatric practice and research. *Psychiatry Research*, 28(2): 193–213.

40. Goelema, M., Regis, M., Haakma, R., *et al.* (2019). Determinants of perceived sleep quality in normal sleepers. *Behavioral Sleep Medicine*, 17: 388–397.

41. Hermans, L.W.A., van Gilst, M.M., Regis, M., *et al.* (2020). Modeling sleep onset misperception in insomnia. *Sleep*, 43(8): zsaa014.

42. Brindle, R.C., Yu, L., Buysse, D.J. & Hall, M.H. (2019). Empirical derivation of cutoff values for the sleep health metric and its relationship to cardiometabolic morbidity: results from the Midlife in the United States (MIDUS) study. *Sleep*, 42(9): zsz116.

43. Bonsignore, M.R., Saaresranta, T. & Riha, R.L. (2019). Sex differences in obstructive sleep apnoea. *European Respiratory Review*, 28(154): 190030.

44. Ananth, S. (2021). Sleep apps: current limitations and challenges. *Sleep Science*, 14(1): 83–86.

45. Asgari, Mehrabadi M., Azimi, I., Sarhaddi, F. *et al.* (2020). Sleep Tracking of a Commercially Available Smart Ring and Smartwatch Against Medical-Grade Actigraphy in Everyday Settings: Instrument Validation Study. *JMIR mHealth and uHealth*, 8(10): e20465.

46. Keklund, G. & Akerstedt, T. (1997). Objective components of individual differences in subjective sleep quality. *Journal of Sleep Research*, 6: 217–220.

47. Della, Monica C., Johnsen, S., Atzori, G., Groeger, J. & Dijk, D. (2018). Rapid Eye Movement Sleep, Sleep Continuity and Slow Wave Sleep as Predictors of Cognition, Mood, and Subjective Sleep Quality in Healthy Men and Women, Aged 20-84 Years. *Frontiers in Psychiatry*, 9: 255.

48. Kaplan, K., Hirshman, J., Hernandez, B., *et al.* (2017). When a gold standard isn't so golden: Lack of prediction of subjective sleep quality from sleep polysomnography. *Biological Psychology*, 123: 37–46.

49. Jackowska, M., Ronaldson, A., Brown, J. & Steptoe, A. (2016). Biological and psychological correlates of self-reported and objective sleep measures. *Journal of Psychosomatic Research*, 84: 52–55.

50. Mantua, J., Gravel, N. & Spencer, R.M. (2016). Reliability of sleep measures from four personal health monitoring devices compared to research-based actigraphy and polysomnography. *Sensors (Basel, Switzerland)*, 16(5): 646.

51. Van Den Berg, J.F., Van Rooij, F.J., Vos, H., *et al.* (2008). Disagreement between subjective and actigraphic measures of sleep duration in a population-based study of elderly persons. *Journal of Sleep Research*, 17(3): 295–302.

52. Ekirch, A. (2005). *At day's close: night in times past.* W. W. Norton and Co.

53. Van de Laar, M., Pevernagie, D., Overeem, S. & Van Mierlo, S. (2015). Subjective sleep characteristics in primary insomnia versus insomnia with comorbid anxiety or mood disorder. *Sleep and Biological Rhythms*, 13: 41–48.

54. Kocevska, D., Lysen, T.S., Dotinga, A., *et al.* (2021). Sleep characteristics across the lifespan in 1.1 million people from the Netherlands, United Kingdom and United States: a systematic review and meta-analysis. *Nature Human Behaviour*, 5(1): 113–122.

55. Kerkhof, G. (2017). Epidemiology of sleep and sleep disorders in the Netherlands. *Sleep Medicine*, 30: 229e239.

56. Hirshkowitz, M., Whiton, K., Albert, S.M., *et al.* (2015). National Sleep Foundation's updated sleep duration recommendations: final report. *Sleep Health*, 1(4): 233–243.

57. Matricciani, L., Bin, Y.S., Lallukka, T., *et al.* (2017). Past, present, and future: trends in sleep duration and implications for public health. *Sleep Health*, 3(5): 317–323.

58. Keyes, K.M., Maslowsky, J., Hamilton, A. & Schulenberg, J. (2015). The great sleep recession: changes in sleep duration among US adolescents, 1991–2012. *Pediatrics*, 135(3): 460–468.

59. Singareddy, R., Bixler, E.O. & Vgontzas, A.N. (2010). Fatigue or daytime sleepiness? *Journal of Clinical Sleep Medicine*, 6(4): 405.

60. Ibid.

61. Williams, A., Dzierzewski, J., Griffin, S., Lind, M., Dick, D. & Rybarczyk, B. (2020). Insomnia Disorder and Behaviorally Induced Insufficient Sleep Syndrome: Prevalence and Relationship to Depression in College Students. *Behavioral Sleep Medicine*, 18: 275–286.

62. Kalmbach, D.A., Cuamatzi-Castelan, A.S., Tonnu, C.V., *et al.* (2018). Hyperarousal and sleep reactivity in insomnia: current insights. *Nature and Science of Sleep*, 10: 193–201.

63. Cano, G., Mochizuki, T. & Saper, C.B. (2008). Neural circuitry of stress-induced insomnia in rats. *Journal of Neuroscience*, 28(40): 10167–84.

64. Hill, T., Trinh, H., Wen, M. & Hale, L. (2016). Perceived neighborhood safety and sleep quality: a global analysis of six countries. *Sleep Medicine*, 18: 56–60.

65. Ibid.

66. Kecklund, G., Akerstedt, T. & Lowden, A. (1997). Morning work: effects of early rising on sleep and alertness. *Sleep*, 20(3): 215–223.

67. Kecklund, G. & Akerstedt, T. (2004). Apprehension of the subsequent working day is associated with a low amount of slow wave sleep. *Biological Psychology*, 66(2): 169–176.

68. Ameen, M.S., Heib, D.P.J., Blume, C. & Schabus, M. (2022). The Brain Selectively Tunes to Unfamiliar Voices during Sleep. *Journal of Neuroscience*, 42(9): 1791–1803.

69. Monk, T.H., Buysse, D.J., Carrier, J. & Kupfer, D.J. (2000). Inducing jet-lag in older people: directional asymmetry. *Journal of Sleep Research*, 9(2): 101–116.

70. Dorffner, G., Vitr, M. & Anderer, P. (2015). The effects of aging on sleep architecture in healthy subjects. *Advances in Experimental Medicine and Biology*, 821: 93–100.

71. Ohayon, M.M., Carskadon, M.A., Guilleminault, C. & Vitiello, M.V. (2004). Meta-analysis of quantitative sleep parameters from childhood to old age in healthy individuals: developing normative sleep values across the human lifespan. *Sleep*, 27(7): 1255–1273.

72. Floyd, J.A., Medler, S.M., Ager, J.W. & Janisse, J.J. (2000). Age-related changes in initiation and maintenance of sleep: a meta-analysis. *Research in Nursing & Health*, 23(2): 106–117.

73. Klerman, E.B., Davis, J.B., Duffy, J.F., Dijk, D.J. & Kronauer, R.E. (2004). Older people awaken more frequently but fall back asleep at the same rate as younger people. *Sleep*, 27(4): 793–798.

74. Dorffner, G., Vitr, M. & Anderer, P. (2015). The effects of aging on sleep architecture in healthy subjects. *Advances in Experimental Medicine and Biology*, 821: 93–100.

75. Luo, J., Zhu, G., Zhao, Q., *et al.* (2013). Prevalence and risk factors of poor sleep quality among Chinese elderly in an urban community: results from the Shanghai aging study. *PloS One*, 8(11): e81261.

76. Foley, D.J., Monjan, A., Simonsick, E.M., Wallace, R.B. & Blazer D,G. (1999). Incidence and remission of insomnia among elderly adults: an epidemiologic study of 6,800 persons over three years. *Sleep*, 22(Suppl 2): S366–372.

77. Vitiello, M.V. (2006). Sleep in normal aging. *Sleep Medicine Clinics*, 1(2): 171–176.

78. Ibid.

79. Xu, Q. & Lang, C.P. (2014). Examining the relationship between subjective sleep disturbance and menopause: a systematic review and meta-analysis. *Menopause*, 21(12): 1301–1318.

80. Gervais, N.J., Mong, J.A. & Lacreuse, A. (2017). Ovarian hormones, sleep and cognition across the adult female lifespan: An integrated perspective. *Frontiers in Neuroendocrinology*, 47: 134–153.

81. Ibid.

82. Ibid.

83. Alblooshi, S., Taylor, M. & Gill, N. (2023). Does menopause elevate the risk for developing depression and anxiety? Results from a systematic review. *Australasian Psychiatry*, 31(2): 165–173.

84. Freedman, R.R. (2005). Hot flashes: behavioral treatments, mechanisms, and relation to sleep. *American Journal of Medicine*, 118, Suppl 12B: 124–130.

3. Why Should We Sleep?

1. Deval, J. (1969). *Afin de vivre bel et bien*. A. Michel.

2. Gotthard, G. (2011). Dreams as a constitutive cultural determinant: the example of ancient Egypt. *International Journal of Dream Research*, 4: 24–30.

3. Smith, D.M. (1998). An Athapaskan way of knowing: Chippewayan ontology. *American Ethnologist*, 25: 412 –432.

4. Schmidt, M. (2014). The energy allocation function of sleep: A unifying theory of sleep, torpor, and continuous wakefulness. *Neuroscience and Biobehavioral Reviews*, 47: 122–153.

5. Jin, Q., Yang, N., Dai, J., *et al.* (2022). Association of sleep duration with all-cause and cardiovascular mortality: A Prospective Cohort Study. *Frontiers in Public Health*, 10: 880276.

6. Li, J., Cao, D., Huang, Y., *et al.* (2022). Sleep duration and health outcomes: an umbrella review. *Sleep and Breathing*, 26(3): 1479–1501.

7. Åkerstedt, T., Ghilotti, F., Grotta, A., Bellavia, A., Lagerros, Y.T. & Bellocco, R. (2017). Sleep duration, mortality and the influence of age. *European Journal of Epidemiology*, 32(10): 881–891.

8. Schmidt, M. (2014). The energy allocation function of sleep: A unifying theory of sleep, torpor, and continuous wakefulness. *Neuroscience and Biobehavioral Reviews*, 47: 122–153.

9. Gao, C., Guo, J., Gong, T.T., *et al.* (2022). Sleep duration/quality with health outcomes: an umbrella review of meta-analyses of prospective studies. *Frontiers in Medicine (Lausanne)*, 8: 813943.

10. Jike, M., Itani, O., Watanabe, N., Buysse, D.J. & Kaneita, Y. (2018). Long sleep duration and health outcomes: A systematic review,

meta-analysis and meta-regression. *Sleep Medicine Reviews*, 39: 25–36.

11. Watanabe, D., Yoshida, T., Watanabe, Y., Yamada, Y., Miyachi, M. & Kimura, M. (2022). Combined use of sleep quality and duration is more closely associated with mortality risk among older adults: a population-based Kyoto-Kameoka prospective cohort study. *Journal of Epidemiology*, 33(12): 591–599.

12. Lovato, N. & Lack, L. (2019). Insomnia and mortality: a meta-analysis. *Sleep Medicine Reviews*, 43: 71-83.

13. Ge, X., Han, F., Huang, Y., *et al.* (2013). Is obstructive sleep apnea associated with cardiovascular and all-cause mortality? *PLoS One*, 8(7): e69432.

14. Lechat, B., Appleton, S., Melaku, Y.A., *et al.* (2022). Comorbid insomnia and sleep apnoea is associated with all-cause mortality. *European Respiratory Journal*, 60(1): 2101958.

15. Brink-Kjaer, A., Leary, E.B., Sun, H., *et al.* (2022). Age estimation from sleep studies using deep learning predicts life expectancy. *npj Digital Medicine*, 5(1): 103.

16. Gu, F., Han, J., Laden, F., *et al.* (2015). Total and cause-specific mortality of U.S. nurses working rotating night shifts. *American Journal of Preventive Medicine*, 48(3): 241–252.

17. Jørgensen, J.T., Karlsen, S., Stayner, L., Hansen, J. & Andersen, Z.J. (2017). Shift work and overall and cause-specific mortality in the Danish nurse cohort. *Scandinavian Journal of Work, Environment & Health*, 43(2): 117–126.

18. Hannerz, H., Soll-Johanning, H., Larsen, A.D. & Garde, A.H. (2019). Night-time work and all-cause mortality in the general working population of Denmark. *International Archives of Occupational and Environmental Health*, 92(4): 577–585.

19. Åkerstedt, T., Narusyte, J. & Svedberg, P. (2020). Night work, mortality, and the link to occupational group and sex. *Scandinavian Journal of Work, Environment & Health*, 46(5): 508–515.

20. Ekirch, A. (2005). *At day's close: night in times past.* W. W. Norton and Co.

21. Katz, L.C., Just, R. & Castell, D.O. (1994). Body position affects recumbent postprandial reflux. *Journal of Clinical Gastroenterology*, 18(4): 280–283.

22. Leung, R.S., Bowman, M.E., Parker, J.D., Newton, G.E. & Bradley, T.D. (2003). Avoidance of the left lateral decubitus position during sleep in patients with heart failure: relationship to cardiac size and function. *Journal of the American College of Cardiology*, 41(2): 227–230.

23. Kohyama, J. (2021). Which is More important for health: sleep quantity or sleep quality? *Children (Basel)*, 8(7): 542.

24. Spiegel, K., Leproult, R., L'hermite-Balériaux, M., Copinschi, G., Penev, P.D. & Van Cauter, E. (2004). Leptin levels are dependent on sleep duration: relationships with sympathovagal balance, carbohydrate regulation, cortisol, and thyrotropin. *Journal of Clinical Endocrinology & Metabolism*, 89(11): 5762–5771.

25. Ismailogullari, S., Bolattürk, O.F., Karaca, Z., *et al.* (2017). Dynamic evaluation of the hypothalamic–pituitary–adrenal and growth hormone axes and metabolic consequences in chronic insomnia; a case–control study. *Sleep and Biological Rhythms*, 15: 317–326.

26. Chan, W.S., Levsen, M.P. & McCrae, C.S. (2018). A meta-analysis of associations between obesity and insomnia diagnosis and symptoms. *Sleep Medicine Reviews*, 40: 170–182.

27. St-Onge, M.P. (2017). Sleep-obesity relation: underlying mechanisms and consequences for treatment. *Obesity Reviews*, 18, Suppl 1: 34–39.

28. Liew, S.C. & Aung, T. (2021). Sleep deprivation and its association with diseases: a review. *Sleep Medicine*, 77: 192–204.

29. Lanfranchi, P.A., Pennestri, M.H., Fradette, L., Dumont, M., Morin, C.M. & Montplaisir, J. (2009). Nighttime blood pressure in normotensive subjects with chronic insomnia: implications for cardiovascular risk. *Sleep*, 32(6): 760–766.

30. Li, L., Gan, Y., Zhou, X., *et al.* (2021). Insomnia and the risk of hypertension: A meta-analysis of prospective cohort studies. *Sleep Medicine Reviews*, 56: 101403.

31. Expert Committee on the Diagnosis and Classification of Diabetes Mellitus (2000). Report of the Expert Committee on the Diagnosis and Classification of Diabetes Mellitus. *Diabetes Care*, 23 Suppl 1: S4–19.

32. Donga, E., Van Dijk, M., Van Dijk, J.G., *et al.* (2010). A single night of partial sleep deprivation induces insulin resistance in multiple metabolic pathways in healthy subjects. Journal of Clinical Endocrinology & Metabolism, 95(6): 2963–2968.

33. Engeda, J., Mezuk, B., Ratliff, S. & Ning, Y. (2013). Association between duration and quality of sleep and the risk of pre-diabetes: evidence from NHANES. *Diabetic Medicine*, 30(6): 676–680.

34. Kowall, B., Lehnich, A.T., Strucksberg, K.H., *et al.* (2016). Associations among sleep disturbances, nocturnal sleep duration, daytime napping, and incident pre-diabetes and type 2 diabetes: the Heinz Nixdorf Recall Study. *Sleep Medicine*, 21: 35–41.

35. Vgontzas, A.N., Liao, D., Pejovic, S., *et al.* (2009). Insomnia with objective short sleep duration is associated with type 2 diabetes: a population-based study. *Diabetes Care*, 32(11): 1980–1985.

36. Kritikou, I., Gehrman, P.R., Mazzotti, D.R. & Chakravorty, S. (2020). Insomnia symptoms with subjective short sleep duration in a random sample from the United Kingdom. *Primary Care Companion for CNS Disorders*, 22(6): 19br02585.

37. Li, Y., Zhang, X., Winkelman, J.W., *et al.* (2014). Association between insomnia symptoms and mortality: a prospective study of U.S. men. *Circulation*, 129(7): 737–746.

38. Schwartz, S.W., Cornoni-Huntley, J., Cole, S.R., *et al.* (1998). Are sleep complaints an independent risk factor for myocardial infarction? *Annals of Epidemiology*, 8(6): 384–392.

39. Thurston, R.C., Chang, Y., Kline, C.E., *et al.* (2024). Trajectories of sleep over Midlife and incident cardiovascular disease events in the study of women's health across the nation. *Circulation*, 149(7): 545–555.

40. Young, T., Finn, L., Austin, D., *et al.* (2003). Menopausal status and sleep-disordered breathing in the Wisconsin Sleep Cohort Study. *American Journal of Respiratory and Critical Care Medicine*, 167: 1181–1185.

41. Ibid.

42. Shi, T., Min, M., Sun, C., Zhang, Y., Liang, M. & Sun, Y. (2020). Does insomnia predict a high risk of cancer? A systematic review and meta-analysis of cohort studies. *Journal of Sleep Research*, 29(1): e12876.

43. Gary, K.A., Winokur, A., Douglas, S.D., Kapoor, S., Zaugg, L. & Dinges, D.F. (1996). Total sleep deprivation and the thyroid axis: effects of sleep and waking activity. *Aviation, Space, and Environmental Medicine*, 67(6): 513–519.

44. Shi, T., Min, M., Sun, C., Zhang, Y., Liang, M. & Sun, Y. (2020). Does insomnia predict a high risk of cancer? A systematic review and meta-analysis of cohort studies. *Journal of Sleep Research*, 29(1): e12876.

45. Chen, Y., Tan, F., Wei, L., *et al.* (2018). Sleep duration and the risk of cancer: a systematic review and meta-analysis including dose-response relationship. *BMC Cancer*, 18(1): 1149.

46. Westermann, J., Lange, T., Textor, J. & Born, J. (2015). System consolidation during sleep – a common principle underlying psychological and immunological memory formation. *Trends in Neuroscience*, 38: 585–597.

47. Prather, A. & Leung, C. (2016). Association of insufficient sleep with respiratory infection among adults in the United States. *JAMA Internal Medicine*, 176: 850–852.

48. Lange, T., Dimitrov, S., Bollinger, T., Diekelmann, S. & Born, J. (2011). Sleep after vaccination boosts immunological memory. *Journal of Immunology*, 187: 283–290.

49. Cermakian, N., Lange, T., Golombek, D., *et al.* (2013). Crosstalk between the circadian clock circuitry and the immune system. *Chronobiology International,* 30(7): 870–888.

50. Takita, E., Yokota, S., Tahara, Y., *et al.* (2013). Biological clock dysfunction exacerbates contact hypersensitivity in mice. *British Journal of Dermatology,* 168(1): 39–46.

51. Dua, S., Ruiz-Garcia, M., Bond, S., *et al.* (2019). Effect of sleep deprivation and exercise on reaction threshold in adults with peanut allergy: a randomized controlled study. *Journal of Allergy and Clinical Immunology,* 144(6): 1584–1594.e2.

52. Lucassen, E.A., De Mutsert, R., Le Cessie, S., *et al.* (2017). NEO study group. Poor sleep quality and later sleep timing are risk factors for osteopenia and sarcopenia in middle-aged men and women: The NEO study. *PLoS One.* 12(5): e0176685.

53. Cedernaes, J., Schönke, M., Westholm, J.O., *et al.* (2018). Acute sleep loss results in tissue-specific alterations in genome-wide DNA methylation state and metabolic fuel utilization in humans. *Science Advances,* 4(8): eaar8590.

54. Zhang, H., Liang, J. & Chen, N. (2020). Do not neglect the role of circadian rhythm in muscle atrophy. *Ageing Research Reviews,* 63: 101155.

55. Lamon, S., Morabito, A., Arentson-Lantz, E., *et al.* (2021). The effect of acute sleep deprivation on skeletal muscle protein synthesis and the hormonal environment. *Physiological Reports,* 9(1): e14660.

56. Areta, J.L., Burke, L.M., Camera, D.M., *et al.* (2014). Reduced resting skeletal muscle protein synthesis is rescued by resistance exercise and protein ingestion following short-term energy deficit. *American Journal of Physiology-Endocrinology Metabolism,* 306(8): E989–997.

57. Tipton, K.D. & Wolfe, R.R. (2001). Exercise, protein metabolism, and muscle growth. *International Journal of Sport Nutrition and Exercise Metabolism,* 11(1): 109–132.

58. Lamon, S., Morabito, A., Arentson-Lantz, E., *et al.* (2021). The effect of acute sleep deprivation on skeletal muscle protein synthesis and the hormonal environment. *Physiological Reports*, 9(1): e14660.

59. Rusch, H., Guardado, P., Baxter, T., Mysliwiec, V. & Gill, J. (2015). Improved sleep quality is associated with reductions in depression and PTSD arousal symptoms and increases in IGF-1 concentrations. *Journal of Clinical Sleep Medicine*, 11: 615–623.

60. Chen, Y., Cui, Y., Chen, S. & Wu, Z. (2017). Relationship between sleep and muscle strength among Chinese university students: a cross-sectional study. *Journal of Musculoskeletal and Neuronal Interactions*, 17: 327–333.

61. Ibid.

62. Pana, A., Sourtzi, P., Kalokairinou, A., Pastroudis, A., Chatzopoulos, S.T. & Velonaki, V.S. (2021). Association between muscle strength and sleep quality and duration among middle-aged and older adults: a systematic review. *European Geriatric Medicine*, 12(1): 27–44.

63. Lucassen, E.A., De Mutsert, R., Le Cessie, S., *et al.* (2017). NEO study group. Poor sleep quality and later sleep timing are risk factors for osteopenia and sarcopenia in middle-aged men and women: The NEO study. *PLoS One*. 12(5): e0176685.

64. Roizenblatt, S., Souza, A.L., Palombini, L., Godoy, L.M., Tufik, S. & Bittencourt, L.R. (2015). Musculoskeletal pain as a marker of health quality. Findings from the Epidemiological Sleep Study among the adult population of Sao Paulo City. *PLoS One*, 10 (11): e0142726.

65. Finan, P.H., Goodin, B.R. & Smith, M.T. (2013). The association of sleep and pain: an update and a path forward. *Journal of Pain*, 14(12): 1539–1552.

66. Husak, A.J. & Bair, M.J. (2020). Chronic pain and sleep disturbances: a pragmatic review of their relationships, comorbidities, and treatments. *Pain Medicine*, 21(6): 1142–1152.

67. Cheatle, M.D., Foster, S., Pinkett, A., Lesneski, M., Qu, D. & Dhingra, L. (2016). Assessing and managing sleep disturbance in patients with chronic pain. *Anesthesiology Clinics*, 34(2): 379–393.

68. Curatolo, M., Müller, M., Ashraf, A., *et al.* (2015). Pain hypersensitivity and spinal nociceptive hypersensitivity in chronic pain: prevalence and associated factors. *Pain*, 156(11): 2373–2382.

69. Tang, N.K., Wright, K.J. & Salkovskis, P.M. (2007). Prevalence and correlates of clinical insomnia co-occurring with chronic back pain. *Journal of Sleep Research*, 16(1): 85–95.

70. Ebbinghaus, H. (1885). *Über das Gedächtnis: Untersuchungen zur experimentellen Psychologie.* Duncker & Humblot.

71. Lee, A. & Wilson, M. (2002). Memory of sequential experience in the hippocampus during slow wave sleep. *Neuron*, 36: 1183–1194.

72. Mednick, S., Nakayama, K. & Stickgold, R. (2003). Sleep-dependent learning: a nap is as good as a night. *Nature Neuroscience*, 6: 697–698.

73. Ibid.

74. Gustavsson, A., Norton, N., Fast, T., *et al.* (2023). Global estimates on the number of persons across the Alzheimer's disease continuum. *Alzheimer's & Dementia*, 19(2): 658–670.

75. Andrade, A.G., Bubu, O.M., Varga, A.W. & Osorio, R.S. (2018). The relationship between obstructive sleep apnea and Alzheimer's Disease. *Journal of Alzheimer's Disease*, 64(s1): S255–S270.

76. Baek, M.S., Han, K., Kwon, H.S., Lee, Y.H., Cho, H. & Lyoo, C.H. (2021). Risks and prognoses of Alzheimer's Disease and vascular dementia in patients with insomnia: a nationwide population-based study. *Frontiers in Neurology*, 12: 611446.

77. Shash, D., Kurth, T., Bertrand, M., *et al.* (2016). Benzodiazepine, psychotropic medication, and dementia: a population-based cohort study. *Alzheimer's & Dementia*, 12: 604–613.

78. He, Q., Chen, X., Wu, T., Li, L. & Fei, X.J.J. (2019). Risk of dementia in long-term benzodiazepine users: evidence from a meta-analysis of observational studies. *Journal of Clinical Neurology*, 15: 9–19.

79. Chen, P.L., Lee, W.J., Sun, W.Z., Oyang, Y.J. & Fuh, J.L. (2012). Risk of dementia in patients with insomnia and long-term use of hypnotics: a population-based retrospective cohort study. *PLoS One*, 7(11): e49113.

80. De Almondes, K.M., Costa, M.V., Malloy-Diniz, L.F. & Diniz, B.S. (2016). Insomnia and risk of dementia in older adults: systematic review and meta-analysis. *Journal of Psychiatric Research*, 77: 109–115.

81. Dotson, V.M., Resnick, S.M. & Zonderman, A.B. (2008). Differential association of concurrent, baseline, and average depressive symptoms with cognitive decline in older adults. *American Journal of Geriatric Psychiatry*, 16: 318–330.

82. Cahill, L., Babinsky, R., Markowitsch, H.J. & McGaugh, J.L. (1995). The amygdala and emotional memory. *Nature*, 377(6547): 295–296.

83. Cha, H., Kim, S., Kim, H., Kim, G. & Kwon, K.Y. (2022). Effect of intensive olfactory training for cognitive function in patients with dementia. *Geriatrics & Gerontology International*, 22(1): 5–11.

84. Oleszkiewicz, A., Abriat, A., Doelz, G., Azema, E. & Hummel, T. (2021). Beyond olfaction: beneficial effects of olfactory training extend to aging-related cognitive decline. *Behavioral Neuroscience*, 135(6): 732–740.

85. Woo, C.C., Miranda, B., Sathishkumar, M., Dehkordi-Vakil, F., Yassa, M.A. & Leon, M. (2023). Overnight olfactory enrichment using an odorant diffuser improves memory and modifies the uncinate fasciculus in older adults. *Frontiers in Neuroscience*, 17: 1200448

86. Artemidorus, D. (1990). *The interpretation of dreams (Oneirocritica)* (translated by R. White), 2nd ed. Noyes Press.

87. Baylor, G. (2001). What do we really know about Mendeleev's dream of the Periodic Table? A note on dreams of scientific problem solving. *Dreaming*, 11: 89–92.

88. Biello, D. (2006). 'Fact or Fiction: Archimedes coined the term "Eureka" in the Bath'. Scientific American.com: https://www.scientificamerican.com/article/fact-or-fiction-archimede/

89. Becchetti, A. & Amadeo, A. (2016). Why we forget our dreams: acetylcholine and norepinephrine in wakefulness and REM sleep. *Behavioral and Brain Sciences*, 39: e202.

90. Lewis, P.A., Knoblich, G. & Poe, G. (2018). How memory replay in sleep boosts creative problem-solving. *Trends in Cognitive Sciences*, 22(6): 491–503.

91. Wagner, U., Gais, S., Haide,r H., Verleger, R. & Born, J. (2004). Sleep inspires insight. *Nature*, 27: 352–355.

92. Ritter, S., Strick, M., Bos, M., Van Baaren, R. & Dijksterhuis, A. (2012). Good morning creativity: task reactivation during sleep enhances beneficial effect of sleep on creative performance. *Journal of Sleep Research*, 21: 643–647.

93. Corsi-Cabrera, M., Velasco, F., Del Río-Portilla, Y., *et al.* (2016). Human amygdala activation during rapid eye movements of rapid eye movement sleep: an intracranial study. *Journal of Sleep Research*, 25(5): 576–582.

94. De Voogd, L.D., Kanen, J.W., Neville, D.A., Roelofs, K., Fernández, G. & Hermans, E.J. (2018). Eye-movement intervention enhances extinction via amygdala deactivation. *Journal of Neuroscience*, 38(40): 8694–8706.

95. Samson, D.R., Clerget, A., Abbas, N., *et al.* (2023). Evidence for an emotional adaptive function of dreams: a cross-cultural study. *Scientific Reports*, 13(1): 16530.

96. Ibid.

97. Gotthard, G. (2011). Dreams as a constitutive cultural determinant: the example of ancient Egypt. *International Journal of Dream Research*, 4: 24–30.

98. Freud, S. (1950 edition; first published 1900). *The interpretation of dreams*. Random House.

99. Baran, B., Pace-Schott, E., Ericson, C. & Spencer, R. (2012). Processing of emotional reactivity and emotional memory over sleep. *Journal of Neuroscience*, 32: 1035e42.

100. Tempesta, D., De Gennaro, L., Natale, V. & Ferrara, M. (2015). Emotional memory processing is influenced by sleep quality. *Sleep Medicine*, 16: 862e70.

101. Huck, N., Mcbride, S., Kendall, A., Grugle, N. & Killgore, W. (2008). The effects of modafinil, caffeine, and dextroamphetamine on judgments of simple versus complex emotional expressions following sleep deprivation. *International Journal of Neuroscience*, 118: 487e502.

102. Tubbs, A.S., Fernandez, F.X., Grandner, M.A., Perlis, M.L. & Klerman, E.B. (2022). The mind after midnight: nocturnal wakefulness, behavioral dysregulation, and psychopathology. *Frontiers in Network Physiology*, 1: 830338.

103. Tubbs, A.S., Perlis, M.L., Basner, M., *et al.* (2020). Relationship of nocturnal wakefulness to suicide risk across months and methods of suicide. *Journal of Clinical Psychiatry*, 81(2): 19m12964.

104. Tononi, G. & Cirelli, C. (2020). Sleep and synaptic down-selection. *European Journal of Neuroscience*, 51(1): 413–421.

105. Hertenstein, E., Feige, B., Gmeiner, T., *et al.* (2019). Insomnia as a predictor of mental disorders: a systematic review and meta-analysis. *Sleep Medicine Reviews*, 43: 96–105.

106. Werner, G.G., Riemann, D. & Ehring, T. (2021). Fear of sleep and trauma-induced insomnia: a review and conceptual model. *Sleep Medicine Reviews*, 55: 101383.

107. Perogamvros, L., Castelnovo, A., Samson, D. & Dang-Vu, T.T. (2020). Failure of fear extinction in insomnia: an evolutionary perspective. *Sleep Medicine Reviews*, 51: 101277.

108. Nutt, D., Wilson, S. & Paterson, L. (2008). Sleep disorders as core symptoms of depression. *Dialogues in Clinical Neuroscience*, 10(3): 329–336.

109. Breslau, N., Roth, T., Rosenthal, L. & Andreski, P. (1996). Sleep disturbance and psychiatric disorders: a longitudinal epidemiological study of young adults. *Biological Psychiatry*, 39: 411–418.

110. Riemann, D., Spiegelhalder, K., Feige, B., Voderholzer, U., Berger, M., Perlis, M., *et al.* (2010). The hyperarousal model of insomnia: a review of the concept and its evidence. *Sleep Medicine Reviews*, 14: 19–31.

111. Strawbridge, R., Young, A.H. & Cleare, A.J. (2017). Biomarkers for depression: recent insights, current challenges and future prospects. *Neuropsychiatric Disease and Treatment*, 13: 1245–1262.

112. Pesonen, A.K., Gradisar, M., Kuula, L., *et al.* (2018). REM sleep fragmentation associated with depressive symptoms and genetic risk for depression in a community-based sample of adolescents. *Journal of Affective Disorders*, 245: 757–763.

113. Riemann, D. & Nissen, C. (2012). Sleep and psychotropic drugs. In: C.M. Morin & C.A. Espie (eds.) *The Oxford Handbook of Sleep and Sleep Disorders*. Oxford University Press.

114. Pesonen, A.K., Gradisar, M., Kuula, L., *et al.* (2018). REM sleep fragmentation associated with depressive symptoms and genetic risk for depression in a community-based sample of adolescents. *Journal of Affective Disorders*, 245: 757–763.

115. Van Someren, E.J.W. (2021). Brain mechanisms of insomnia: new perspectives on causes and consequences. *Physiological Reviews*, 101(3): 995–1046.

116. Ioannou, M., Wartenberg, C., Greenbrook, J.T.V., *et al.* (2021). Sleep deprivation as treatment for depression: systematic review and meta-analysis. *Acta Psychiatrica Scandinavica*, 143(1): 22–35.

117. Okechukwu, C.E., Colaprico, C., Di Mario, S., *et al.* (2023). The relationship between working night shifts and depression among nurses: a systematic review and meta-analysis. *Healthcare (Basel)*, 11(7): 937.

4. Sleepless Nights

1. Beausacq, M., Beausacq, D. & Prudhomme, S. (1883). *Maximes de la vie*. Paris.

2. Yetish, G., Kaplan, H., Gurven, M., *et al.* (2015). Natural sleep and its seasonal variations in three pre-industrial societies. *Current Biology*, 25: 2862–2868.

3. Morin, C.M. & Jarrin, D.C. (2022). Epidemiology of insomnia: prevalence, course, risk factors, and public health burden. *Sleep Medicine Clinics*, 17(2): 173–191.

4. Zhang, B. & Wing, Y. (2006). Sex differences in insomnia: a meta-analysis. *Sleep*, 29: 85–93.

5. American Academy of Sleep Medicine. (2014). *The International Classification of Sleep Disorders – Third Edition* (*ICSD-3*). American Academy of Sleep Medicine.

6. Spielman, A. & Glovinsky, P. (1991). The varied nature of insomnia. In P. Hauri (ed.) *Case Studies in Insomnia*. Plenum Press.

7. Hofmann, S.G., Ellard, K.K. & Siegle, G.J. (2012). Neurobiological correlates of cognitions in fear and anxiety: a cognitive-neurobiological information-processing model. *Cognition and Emotion*, 26(2): 282–299.

8. Ibid.

9. Thomsen, D., Yung Mehlsen, M., Christensen, S. & Zachariae, R. (2003). Rumination, relationship with negative mood and sleep quality. *Personality and Individual Differences*, 34: 1293–1301.

10. Nolen-Hoeksema, S., Larson, J. & Grayson, C. (1999). Explaining the gender difference in depressive symptoms. *Journal of Personality and Social Psychology*, 77: 1061–1072.

11. Merikangas, K., He, J., Burstein, M., *et al.* (2010). Lifetime prevalence of mental disorders in U.S. adolescents: results from the National Comorbidity Survey Replication--Adolescent Supplement (NCS-A). *Journal of the American Academy of Child and Adolescent Psychiatry*, 49: 980–989.

12. Wang, J., Korczykowski, M., Rao, H., *et al.* (2007). Gender difference in neural response to psychological stress. *Social Cognitive and Affective Neuroscience*, 2: 227–239.

13. Wuyts, J., De Valck, E., Vandekerckhove, M., *et al.* (2012). The influence of pre-sleep cognitive arousal on sleep onset processes. *International Journal of Psychophysiology*, 83(1): 8–15.

14. Baglioni, C., Spiegelhalder, K., Lombardo, C. & Riemann, D. (2010). Sleep and emotions: a focus on insomnia. *Sleep Medicine Reviews*, 14(4):227-38.

15. Bonnet, M.H. & Arand, D.L. (2003). Situational insomnia: consistency, predictors, and outcomes. *Sleep.* 26(8): 1029–1036.

16. Drake, C., Richardson, G., Roehrs, T., Scofield H. & Roth, T. (2004). Vulnerability to stress-related sleep disturbance and hyperarousal. *Sleep.* 27(2): 285–291.

17. Bonnet, M.H. & Arand, D.L. (2003). Situational insomnia: consistency, predictors, and outcomes. *Sleep.* 26(8): 1029–1036.

18. Jarrin, D.C., Chen, I.Y., Ivers, H. & Morin, C.M. (2014). The role of vulnerability in stress-related insomnia, social support and coping styles on incidence and persistence of insomnia. *Journal of Sleep Research*, 23(6): 681–688.

19. Drake, C.L., Scofield, H. & Roth, T. (2008). Vulnerability to insomnia: the role of familial aggregation. *Sleep Medicine*, 9(3): 297–302.

20. Fernandez-Mendoza, J., Shaffer, M.L., Olavarrieta-Bernardino, S., *et al.* (2014). Cognitive-emotional hyperarousal in the offspring of parents vulnerable to insomnia: a nuclear family study. *Journal of Sleep Research*, 23(5): 489–498.

21. Kalmbach, D.A., Pillai, V., Arnedt, J.T., Anderson, J.R. & Drake, C.L. (2016). Sleep system sensitization: evidence for changing roles of etiological factors in insomnia. *Sleep Medicine*, 21: 63–69.

22. Reffi, A.N., Kalmbach, D.A., Cheng, P., *et al.* (2022). Sleep reactivity as a potential pathway from childhood abuse to adult insomnia. *Sleep Medicine*, 94: 70–75.

23. Park, K., Kim, G., Lee, J. & Suh, S. (2023). Differences in treatment effects of cognitive-behavioral therapy for insomnia based on sleep reactivity: a preliminary study. *Behavioral Sleep Medicine*, 21(3): 332–343.

24. Yang, L., Zhang, J., Luo, X., *et al.* (2023). Effectiveness of one-week internet-delivered cognitive behavioral therapy for insomnia topre-vent progression from acute to chronic insomnia: A two-arm, multi-center, randomized controlled trial. *Psychiatry Research*, 321: 115066.

25. Insana, S.P., Kolko, D.J. & Germain, A. (2012). Early-life trauma is associated with rapid eye movement sleep fragmentation among military veterans. *Biological Psychology*, 89(3): 570–579.

26. Glod, C.A., Teicher, M.H., Hartman, C.R. & Harakal, T. (1997). Increased nocturnal activity and impaired sleep maintenance in abused children. *Journal of the American Academy of Child & Adolescent Psychiatry*, 36(9): 1236–1243.

27. Maurer, L.F., Sharman, R., Espie, C.A. & Kyle, S.D. (2024). The effect of sleep restriction therapy for insomnia on REM sleep fragmentation: A secondary analysis of a randomised controlled trial. *Journal of Sleep Research*, 33(1): e13982.

28. Van de Laar, M., Pevernagie, D., Van Mierlo, P. & Overeem, S. (2015). Psychiatric comorbidity and aspects of cognitive coping negatively predict outcome in cognitive behavioral treatment of psychophysiological insomnia. *Behavioral Sleep Medicine*, 13: 140–156.

29. Ibid.

30. Gebara, M.A., Siripong, N., DiNapoli, E.A., *et al.* (2018). Effect of insomnia treatments on depression: a systematic review and meta-analysis. *Depression and Anxiety*, 35(8): 717–731.

31. Van de Laar, M., Verbeek, I., Pevernagie, D., Aldenkamp, A. & Overeem, S. (2010). The role of personality traits in insomnia. *Sleep Medicine Reviews*, 14: 61–68.

32. Ibid.

33. Lundh, L., Broman, J. & Hetta, J. (1995). Personality traits in patients with persistent insomnia. *Personality and Individual Differences*, 18: 393–403.

34. Van de Laar, M., Leufkens, T., Bakker, B., Pevernagie, D. & Overeem, S. (2017). Phenotypes of sleeplessness: stressing the need for psychodiagnostics in the assessment of insomnia. *Psychology, Health and Medicine*, 22: 902–910.

5. The Primal Basics

1. Hesse, H. (1943). *Das Glasperlenspiel*. Fretz & Wasmuth.

2. Samson, D.R., Crittenden, A.N., Mabulla, I.A., *et al.* (2017). Hadza sleep biology: Evidence for flexible sleep-wake patterns in hunter-gatherers. *American Journal of Physical Anthropology*, 162(3): 573–582.

3. Hippocrates, 'Regimen in acute diseases' (translated by Chadwick J., Lonie, I. & Mann W.) in G. Loyd (ed.) (1983) *Hippocratic writings*. Penguin.

4. Hudson, A.N., Van Dongen, H.P.A. & Honn, K.A. (2020). Sleep deprivation, vigilant attention, and brain function: a review. *Neuropsychopharmacology*, 45(1): 21–30.

5. Pires, G.N., Bezerra, A.G., Tufik, S. & Andersen, M.L. (2016). Effects of acute sleep deprivation on state anxiety levels: a systematic review and meta-analysis. *Sleep Medicine*, 24: 109–118.

6. Kuna, S.T., Maislin, G., Pack, F.M., *et al.* (2012). Heritability of performance deficit accumulation during acute sleep deprivation in twins. *Sleep*. 35(9): 1223–1233.

7. Putilov, A.A., Donskaya, O.G., Poluektov, M.G. & Dorokhov, V.B. (2021). Age- and gender-associated differences in the sleepy brain's electroencephalogram. *Physiological Measurement*, 42(4).

8. Gharibi, V., Mokarami, H., Cousins, R., Jahangiri, M. & Eskandari, D. (2020). Excessive daytime sleepiness and safety performance:

comparing proactive and reactive approaches. *International Journal of Occupational and Environmental Medicine*, 11(2): 95–107.

9. Roehrs, T., Shore, E., Papineau, K., Rosenthal, L. & Roth, T. (1996). A two-week sleep extension in sleepy normals. *Sleep*, 19(7): 576–582.

10. Harrison, Y. & Horne, J.A. (1996). Long-term extension to sleep: are we really chronically sleep deprived? *Psychophysiology*, 33(1): 22–30.

11. Blume, C., Schmidt, M.H. & Cajochen, C. (2020). Effects of the COVID-19 lockdown on human sleep and rest-activity rhythms. *Current Biology*, 30(14): R795–R797.

12. Wright, K.P. Jr, Linton, S.K., Withrow, D., *et al.* (2020). Sleep in university students prior to and during COVID-19 Stay-at-Home orders. *Current Biology*, 30(14): R797–R798.

13. Cellini, N., Canale, N., Mioni, G. & Costa, S. (2020). Changes in sleep pattern, sense of time and digital media use during COVID-19 lockdown in Italy. *Journal of Sleep Research*, 29(4): e13074.

14. Bottary, R., Simonelli, G., Cunningham, T.J., Kensinger, E.A. & Mantua, J. (2020). Sleep extension: an explanation for increased pandemic dream recall? *Sleep*, 43(11): zsaa131.

15. Elhami, Athar M., Atef-Vahid, M.K. & Ashouri, A. (2020). The influence of shift work on the quality of sleep and executive functions. *Journal of Circadian Rhythms*, 18: 4.

16. Booker, L.A., Magee, M., Rajaratnam, S.M.W., Sletten, T.L. & Howard, M.E. (2018). Individual vulnerability to insomnia, excessive sleepiness and shift work disorder amongst healthcare shift workers: a systematic review. *Sleep Medicine Reviews*, 41: 220–233.

17. Storemark, S.S., Fossum, I.N., Bjorvatn, B., Moen, B.E., Flo, E. & Pallesen, S. (2013). Personality factors predict sleep-related shift work tolerance in different shifts at 2-year follow-up: a prospective study. *British Medical Journal Open*. 3(11): e003696.

18. Wittmann, M., Dinich, J., Merrow, M. & Roenneberg T. (2006). Social jetlag: misalignment of biological and social time. *Chronobiology International*, 23(1–2): 497–509.

19. Vallat, R., Berry, S.E., Tsereteli, N., *et al.* (2022). How people wake up is associated with previous night's sleep together with physical activity and food intake. *Nature Communications*, 13(1): 7116.

20. Samson, D.R., Crittenden, A.N., Mabulla, I.A., *et al.* (2017). Hadza sleep biology: Evidence for flexible sleep-wake patterns in hunter-gatherers. *American Journal of Physical Anthropology*, 162(3): 573–582.

21. Dutheil, F., Danini, B., Bagheri, R., *et al.* (2021). Effects of a short daytime nap on cognitive performance: a systematic review and meta-analysis. *International Journal of Environmental Research and Public Health*, 18(19): 10212.

22. Farhadian, N., Khazaie, H., Nami, M. & Khazaie, S. (2021). The role of daytime napping in declarative memory performance: a systematic review. *Sleep Medicine*, 84: 134–141.

23. Hołda, M., Głodek, A., Dankiewicz-Berger, M., Skrzypińska, D. & Szmigielska, B. (2020). Ill-defined problem solving does not benefit from daytime napping. *Frontiers in Psychology*, 11: 559.

24. Zion, N. & Shochat, T. (2019). Let them sleep: The effects of a scheduled nap during the night shift on sleepiness and cognition in hospital nurses. *Journal of Advanced Nursing*, 75(11): 2603–2615.

25. Lastella, M., Halson, S.L., Vitale, J.A., Memon, A.R. & Vincent, G.E. (2021). To nap or not to nap? A systematic review evaluating napping behavior in athletes and the impact on various measures of athletic performance. *Nature and Science of Sleep*, 13: 841–862.

26. Stepan, M.E., Altmann, E.M. & Fenn, K.M. (2021). Slow-wave sleep during a brief nap is related to reduced cognitive deficits during sleep deprivation. *Sleep*, 44(11): zsab152.

27. Ibid.

28. Ye, L., Hutton Johnson, S., Keane, K., Manasia, M. & Gregas, M. (2015). Napping in college students and its relationship with night-time sleep. *Journal of American College Health*, 63(2): 88–97.

29. Pereira, R., Hartescu, I., Morgan, K., *et al.* (2021). Is daytime napping a risk factor for persistent insomnia symptoms? *Sleep*, 44, S2(323): A129–A130.

30. Jang, K.H., Lee, J.H., Kim, S.J. & Kwon, H.J. (2018). Characteristics of napping in community-dwelling insomnia patients. *Sleep Medicine*, 45: 49–54.

31. Yang, M.J., Zhang, Z., Wang, Y.J., *et al.* (2022). Association of nap frequency with hypertension or ischemic stroke supported by prospective cohort data and Mendelian randomization in predominantly middle-aged European subjects. *Hypertension*, 79(9): 1962–1970.

32. Ogawa, K., Kaizuma-Ueyama,E. & Hayashi, M. (2022). Effects of using a snooze alarm on sleep inertia after morning awakening. *Journal of Physiological Anthropology*, 41(1): 43.

33. Ekstedt, M., Akerstedt, T. & Söderström, M. (2004). Microarousals during sleep are associated with increased levels of lipids, cortisol, and blood pressure. *Psychosomatic Medicine*, 66(6): 925–931.

34. Hilditch, C.J. & McHill, A.W. (2019). Sleep inertia: current insights. *Nature and Science of Sleep*, 11: 155–165.

35. Sundelin, T., Landry, S. & Axelsson, J. (2023). Is snoozing losing? Why intermittent morning alarms are used and how they affect sleep, cognition, cortisol, and mood. *Journal of Sleep Research*, 17: e14054.

36. Samson, D.R., Crittenden, A.N., Mabulla, I.A., *et al.* (2017). Hadza sleep biology: Evidence for flexible sleep-wake patterns in hunter-gatherers. *American Journal of Physical Anthropology*, 162(3): 573–582.

37. Lawrenson, J.G., Hull, C.C. & Downie, L.E. (2017). The effect of blue-light blocking spectacle lenses on visual performance, macular health and the sleep-wake cycle: a systematic review of the literature. *Ophthalmic and Physiological Optics*, 37(6): 644–654.

38. Burkhart, K. & Phelps, J.R. (2009). Amber lenses to block blue light and improve sleep: a randomized trial. *Chronobiology International*, 26(8): 1602–1612.

39. Shechter, A., Kim, E.W., St-Onge, M.P. & Westwood, A.J. (2018). Blocking nocturnal blue light for insomnia: a randomized controlled trial. *Journal of Psychiatric Research*, 96: 196–202.

40. Vagge, A., Ferro, Desideri L., Del Noce, C., Di Mola, I., Sindaco, D. & Traverso, C.E. (2021). Blue light filtering ophthalmic lenses: a systematic review. *Seminars in Ophthalmology*, 36(7): 541–548.

41. Van Kerkhof, L.W.M., Van der Maaden, T., Van der Meijden, W., et al. (2019). Screen use blue light and sleep (Schermgebruik blauw licht en slaap), Rijksinstituut voor Volksgezondheid en Milieu (RIVM).

42. Tähkämö, L., Partonen, T. & Pesonen, A.K. (2019). Systematic review of light exposure impact on human circadian rhythm. *Chronobiology International*, 36(2): 151–170.

43. Arshad, D., Joyia, U.M., Fatima, S., *et al.* (2021). The adverse impact of excessive smartphone screen-time on sleep quality among young adults: a prospective cohort. *Sleep Science*, 14(4): 337–341.

44. Heo, J.Y., Kim, K., Fava, M., *et al.* (2017). Effects of smartphone use with and without blue light at night in healthy adults: a randomized, double-blind, cross-over, placebo-controlled comparison. *Journal of Psychiatric Research*, 87: 61–70.

45. Wood, B., Rea, M.S., Plitnick, B. & Figueiro, M.G. (2013). Light level and duration of exposure determine the impact of self-luminous tablets on melatonin suppression. *Applied Ergonomics*, 44(2): 237–240.

46. Nagare, R., Plitnick, B. & Figueiro, M.G. (2019). Does the iPad night shift mode reduce melatonin suppression? *Lighting Research & Technology*, 51(3): 373–383.

47. Lund, L., Sølvhøj, I.N., Danielsen, D. & Andersen, S. (2021). Electronic media use and sleep in children and adolescents in western countries: a systematic review. *BMC Public Health*, 21(1): 1598.

48. Bauducco, S., Pillion, M., Bartel, K., Reynolds, C., Kahn, M. & Gradisar, M. (2024). A bidirectional model of sleep and technology

use: a theoretical review of how much, for whom, and which mechanisms. *Sleep Medicine Reviews*, 76: 101933.

49. Wams, E.J., Woelders, T., Marring, I., *et al.* (2017). Linking light exposure and subsequent sleep: a field polysomnography study in humans. *Sleep*, 40(12): zsx165

50. Brown, T.M., Brainard, G.C., Cajochen, C., *et al.* (2022). Recommendations for daytime, evening, and nighttime indoor light exposure to best support physiology, sleep, and wakefulness in healthy adults. *PLoS Biology*, 20(3): e3001571.

51. Lok, R., Woelders, T., Gordijn, M.C.M., *et al.* (2022). Bright light during wakefulness improves sleep quality in healthy men: a forced desynchrony study under dim and bright light (III). *Journal of Biological Rhythms*, 37(4): 429–441.

52. Amdisen, L., Daugaard, S., Vestergaard, J.M., *et al.* (2022). A longitudinal study of morning, evening, and night light intensities and nocturnal sleep quality in a working population. *Chronobiology International*, 39(4): 579–589.

53. Rångtell, F.H., Ekstrand, E., Rapp, L., *et al.* (2016). Two hours of evening reading on a self-luminous tablet vs. reading a physical book does not alter sleep after daytime bright light exposure. *Sleep Medicine*, 23: 111–118.

54. Brown, T.M., Brainard, G.C., Cajochen, C., *et al.* (2022). Recommendations for daytime, evening, and nighttime indoor light exposure to best support physiology, sleep, and wakefulness in healthy adults. *PLoS Biology*, 20(3): e3001571.

55. Ibid.

56. Rishi, M.A., Ahmed, O., Barrantes Perez, J.H., *et al.* (2020). Daylight saving time: an American Academy of Sleep Medicine position statement. *Journal of Clinical Sleep Medicine*, 16(10): 1781–1784.

57. Hou, G., Gao, J., Chen, Y., *et al.* (2020). Winter-to-summer seasonal migration of microlithic human activities on the Qinghai-Tibet Plateau. *Scientific Reports*, 10(1): 11659.

58. Yetish, G., Kaplan, H., Gurven, M., *et al.* (2015). Natural sleep and its seasonal variations in three pre-industrial societies. *Current Biology*, 25: 2862–2868.

59. Rishi, M.A., Ahmed, O., Barrantes Perez, J.H., *et al.* (2020). Daylight saving time: an American Academy of Sleep Medicine position statement. *Journal of Clinical Sleep Medicine*, 16(10): 1781–1784.

60. Hashizaki, M., Nakajima, H., Shiga, T., Tsutsumi, M. & Kume, K. (2018). A longitudinal large-scale objective sleep data analysis revealed a seasonal sleep variation in the Japanese population. *Chronobiology International*, 35: 933–945.

61. Mattingly, S.M., Grover, T., Martinez, G.J., *et al.* (2021). The effects of seasons and weather on sleep patterns measured through longitudinal multimodal sensing. *NPJ Digital Medicine*, 4(1): 76.

62. Tsang, T.W., Mui, K.W. & Wong, L.T. (2021). Investigation of thermal comfort in sleeping environment and its association with sleep quality. *Building and Environment*, 187, Article 107406.

63. Harding, E.C., Franks, N.P. & Wisden, W. (2020). Sleep and thermoregulation. *Current Opinion in Physiology*, 15: 7–13.

64. Harding, E.C., Franks, N.P. & Wisden, W. (2019). The temperature dependence of sleep. *Frontiers in Neuroscience*, 13: 336.

65. Gilbert, S.S., Van den Heuvel, C.J., Ferguson, S.A. & Dawson, D. (2004). Thermoregulation as a sleep signalling system. *Sleep Medicine Reviews*, 8: 81–93.

66. Muzet, A., Libert, J.P. & Candas, V. (1984). Ambient temperature and human sleep. *Experientia*, 1984; 40: 425–429.

67. Kräuchi K. (2007). The thermophysiological cascade leading to sleep initiation in relation to phase of entrainment. *Sleep Medicine Reviews*, 11(6), 439–451.

68. Okamoto-Mizuno, K. & Mizuno, K. (2012). Effects of thermal environment on sleep and circadian rhythm. *Journal of Physiological Anthropology*, 31: 14.

69. Haghayegh, S., Khoshnevis, S., Smolensky, M.H., Diller, K.R. & Castriotta, R.J. (2019). Before-bedtime passive body heating by warm shower or bath to improve sleep: a systematic review and meta-analysis. *Sleep Medicine Reviews*, 46: 124–135.

70. Strøm-Tejsen, P., Mathiasen, S., Bach, M. & Petersen, S. (2016). The effects of increased bedroom air temperature on sleep and next-day mental performance. The 14th International Conference of Indoor Air Quality and Climate. Ghent, Belgium: Volume: Paper 640.

71. Joshi, S.S., Lesser, T.J., Olsen, J.W. & O'Hara, B.F. (2016). The importance of temperature and thermoregulation for optimal human sleep. *Energy and Buildings*, 131: 153–157.

72. Liu, Y., Song, C., Wang, Y., Wang, D. & Liu, J. (2014). Experimental study and evaluation of the thermal environment for sleeping. *Building and Environment*, 82: 546–555.

73. Komagata, N., Latifi, B., Rusterholz, T., *et al.* (2019). Dynamic REM sleep modulation by ambient temperature and the critical role of the melanin-concentrating hormone system. *Current Biology*, 29(12): 1976–1987.e4.

74. Joshi, S.S., Lesser, T.J., Olsen, J.W. & O'Hara, B.F. (2016). The importance of temperature and thermoregulation for optimal human sleep. *Energy and Buildings*, 131: 153–157.

75. Minor, K., Bjerre-Nielsen, A., Jonasdottir, S.S., Lehman, S. & Obradovich, N. (2022). Rising temperatures erode sleep globally. *One Earth*, 5: 534–549.

76. Tsuzuki, K., Morito, N. & Nishimiya, H. (2015). Sleep quality and air conditioner use. *Extreme Physiology & Medicine*, 4 (Suppl 1): A129.

77. Samson, D.R., Crittenden, A.N., Mabulla, I.A., *et al.* (2017). Hadza sleep biology: Evidence for flexible sleep-wake patterns in hunter-gatherers. *American Journal of Physical Anthropology*, 162(3): 573–582.

78. Minor, K., Bjerre-Nielsen, A., Jonasdottir, S.S., Lehman, S. & Obradovich, N. (2022). Rising temperatures erode sleep globally. *One Earth*, 5: 534–549.

79. Rifkin, D.I., Long, M.W. & Perry, M.J. (2018). Climate change and sleep: a systematic review of the literature and conceptual framework. *Sleep Medicine Reviews*, 42: 3–9.

80. Herberger, S., Kräuchi, K., Glos, M., *et al.* (2020). Effects of sleep on a high-heat capacity mattress on sleep stages, EEG power spectra, cardiac interbeat intervals and body temperatures in healthy middle-aged men. *Sleep*, 43(5): zsz271.

81. Yim, J. (2015). Optimal pillow conditions for high-quality sleep: a theoretical review. *Indian Journal of Science and Technology*, 8(S5): 135.

82. Lee, H. & Park, S. (2006). Quantitative effects of mattress types (comfortable vs. uncomfortable) on sleep quality through polysomnography and skin temperature. *International Journal of Industrial Ergonomics*, 36(11).

83. Caggiari, G., Talesa, G.R., Toro, G., Jannelli, E., Monteleone, G. & Puddu, L. (2021). What type of mattress should be chosen to avoid back pain and improve sleep quality? Review of the literature. *Journal of Orthopaedics and Traumatology*, 22(1): 51.

84. Radwan, A., Fess, P., James, D., *et al.* (2015). Effect of different mattress designs on promoting sleep quality, pain reduction, and spinal alignment in adults with or without back pain; systematic review of controlled trials. *Sleep Health*, 1(4): 257–267.

85. Chun-Yiu, J.P., Man-Ha, S.T. & Chak-Lun, A.F. (2021). The effects of pillow designs on neck pain, waking symptoms, neck disability, sleep quality and spinal alignment in adults: a systematic review and meta-analysis. *Clinical Biomechanics*, 85: 105353.

86. Shin, M., Halaki, M., Swan, P., Ireland, A.H. & Chow, C.M. (2016). The effects of fabric for sleepwear and bedding on sleep at ambient temperatures of 17°C and 22°C. *Nature and Science of Sleep*, 8: 121–131.

87. Eron, K., Kohnert, L., Watters, A., Logan, C., Weisner-Rose, M. & Mehler, P.S. (2020). Weighted blanket Use: a systematic review. *American Journal of Occupational Therapy*, 74(2): 1–14.

88. Ekholm, B., Spulber, S. & Adler, M. (2020). A randomized controlled study of weighted chain blankets for insomnia in psychiatric disorders. *Journal of Clinical Sleep Medicine*, 16(9): 1567–1577.

89. Tang, N.K., Schmidt D., Harvey & A.G. (2007). Sleeping with the enemy: clock monitoring in the maintenance of insomnia. *Journal of Behavior Therapy and Experimental Psychiatry*, 38(1): 40–55.

90. Dawson, S.C., Krakow, B., Haynes, P.L., Rojo-Wissar, D.M., McIver, N.D. & Ulibarri, V.A. (2023). Use of sleep aids in insomnia: the role of time monitoring behavior. *Primary Care Companion for CNS Disorders*, 25(3): 22m03344.

91. Harvey, A.G. (2002). A cognitive model of insomnia. *Behaviour Research and Therapy*, 40: 869–893.

92. Samson, D.R., Crittenden, A.N., Mabulla, I.A., *et al.* (2017). Hadza sleep biology: Evidence for flexible sleep-wake patterns in hunter-gatherers. *American Journal of Physical Anthropology*, 162(3): 573–582.

93. Xie, Y., Liu, S., Chen, X.J., Yu, H.H., Yang, Y. & Wang, W. (2021). Effects of exercise on sleep quality and insomnia in adults: a systematic review and meta-analysis of randomized controlled trials. *Frontiers in Psychiatry*, 12: 664499.

94. Dolezal, B.A., Neufeld, E.V., Boland, D.M., Martin, J.L. & Cooper, C.B. (2017). Interrelationship between sleep and exercise: a systematic review. *Advanced Preventive Medicine*, 2017(1): 1364387.

95. Ibid.

96. Ezati, M., Keshavarz, M., Barandouzi, Z.A. & Montazeri, A. (2020). The effect of regular aerobic exercise on sleep quality and fatigue among female student dormitory residents. *BMC Sports Science, Medicine and Rehabilitation*, 12: 44.

97. Wang, F. & Boros, S. (2021). The effect of physical activity on sleep quality: a systematic review. *European Journal of Physiotherapy*, 23(1): 11–18.

98. Händel, M.N., Andersen, H.K., Ussing, A., *et al.* (2023). The short-term and long-term adverse effects of melatonin treatment in children and adolescents: a systematic review and GRADE assessment. *EClinicalMedicine*, 61: 102083.

99. Banno, M., Harada, Y., Taniguchi, M., *et al.* (2018). Exercise can improve sleep quality: a systematic review and meta-analysis. *PeerJ*, 6: e5172.

100. Yang, P.Y., Ho, K.H., Chen, H.C. & Chien, M.Y. (2012). Exercise training improves sleep quality in middle-aged and older adults with sleep problems: a systematic review. *Journal of Physiotherapy*, 58(3): 157–163.

101. Lederman, O., Ward, P.B., Firth, J., *et al.* (2019). Does exercise improve sleep quality in individuals with mental illness? A systematic review and meta-analysis. *Journal of Psychiatric Research*, 109: 96–106.

102. Herring, M.P., Kline, C.E. & O'Connor, P.J. (2015). Effects of exercise on sleep among young women with generalized anxiety disorder. *Mental Health and Physical Activity*, 9: 59–66.

103. Frimpong, E., Mograss, M., Zvionow, T. & Dang-Vu, T.T. (2021). The effects of evening high-intensity exercise on sleep in healthy adults: a systematic review and meta-analysis. *Sleep Medicine Reviews*, 60: 101535.

104. Stutz, J., Eiholzer, R. & Spengler, C.M. (2019). Effects of evening exercise on sleep in healthy participants: a systematic review and meta-analysis. *Sports Medicine*, 49(2): 269–287.

105. Ibid.

106. Gupta, L., Morgan, K. & Gilchrist, S. (2017). Does elite sport degrade sleep quality? A systematic review. *Sports Medicine*, 47(7): 1317–1333.

107. Fietze, I., Strauch, J., Holzhausen, M., *et al.* (2009). . Sleep quality in professional ballet dancers. *Chronobiology International*, 26(6): 1249–1262.

108. Ahrberg, K., Dresler, M., Niedermaier, S., Steiger, A. & Genzel, L. (2012). The interaction between sleep quality and academic performance. *Journal of Psychiatric Research*, 46(12): 1618–1622.

109. Juliff, L.E., Halson, S.L. & Peiffer, J.J. (2015). Understanding sleep disturbance in athletes prior to important competitions. *Journal of Science and Medicine in Sport*, 18(1): 13–18.

110. Lastella, M., Roach, G.D., Halson, S.L. & Sargent, C. (2015). Sleep/wake behaviours of elite athletes from individual and team sports. *European Journal of Sport Science*, 15(2): 94–100.

111. Erlacher, D., Ehrlenspiel, F., Adegbesan, O.A. & El-Din, H.G. (2011). Sleep habits in German athletes before important competitions or games. *Journal of Sports Sciences*, 29(8): 859–866.

112. Stephens, T. & Caspersen, C.J. (1994). The demography of physical activity. In: C. Bouchard, R.J. Shephard & T. Stephens (eds) *Physical Activity, Fitness, and Health: International Proceedings and Consensus Statement*. Human Kinetics Publishers: p.204.

113. Barlow, P.W., Mikulecký, M. Sr & Střeštík, J. (2010). Tree-stem diameter fluctuates with the lunar tides and perhaps with geomagnetic activity. *Protoplasma*, 247(1-2): 25–43.

114. Kronfeld-Schor, N., Dominoni, D., De la Iglesia, H., *et al.* (2013). Chronobiology by moonlight. *Proceedings Biological Sciences*, 280(1765): 20123088.

115. Cajochen, C., Altanay-Ekici, S., Münch, M., Frey, S., Knoblauch, V. & Wirz-Justice, A. (2013). Evidence that the lunar cycle influences human sleep. *Current Biology*, 23(15): 1485–1488.

116. Smith, M., Croy I. & Persson Waye, K. Human sleep and cortical reactivity are influenced by lunar phase. *Current Biology*, 24(12): R551–R552.

117. Cordi, M., Ackermann, S., Bes, F.W., *et al.* (2014). Lunar cycle effects on sleep and the file drawer problem. *Current Biology*, 24(12): R549–R550.

118. Casiraghi, L., Spiousas, I., Dunster, G.P., *et al.* (2021). Moonstruck sleep: Synchronization of human sleep with the moon cycle under field conditions. *Science Advances*, 7(5): eabe0465.

119. Walbeek, T.J., Harrison, E.M., Gorman, M.R. & Glickman, G.L. (2021). Naturalistic intensities of light at night: a review of the potent effects of very dim light on circadian responses and considerations for translational research. *Frontiers in Neurology*, 12: 625334.

120. Marlowe, F. *The Hadza: Hunter-Gatherers of Tanzania*. Vol. 3. University of California Press, 2010.

121. Sutanto, C.N., Wang, M.X., Tan, D. & Kim, J.E. (2020). Association of sleep quality and macronutrient distribution: a systematic review and meta-regression. *Nutrients*, 12(1): 126.

122. Zhou, J., Kim, J.E., Armstrong, C.L., Chen, N. & Campbell, W.W. (2016). Higher-protein diets improve indexes of sleep in energy-restricted overweight and obese adults: results from 2 randomized controlled trials. *American Journal of Clinical Nutrition*, 103(3): 766–774.

123. Santana, A.A., Pimentel, G.D., Romualdo, M., *et al.* (2012). Sleep duration in elderly obese patients correlated negatively with intake fatty. *Lipids in Health and Disease*, 11: 99.

124. Sutanto, C.N., Wang, M.X., Tan, D. & Kim, J.E. (2020). Association of sleep quality and macronutrient distribution: a systematic review and meta-regression. *Nutrients*, 12(1): 126.

125. Phillips, F., Chen, C.N., Crisp, A.H., *et al.* (1975). Isocaloric diet changes and electroencephalographic sleep. *The Lancet*, 2(7938): 723–725.

126. Peuhkuri, K., Sihvola, N. & Korpela, R. (2012). Diet promotes sleep duration and quality. *Nutrition Research*, 32(5): 309–319.

127. Iao, S.I., Jansen, E., Shedden, K., *et al.* (2021). Associations between bedtime eating or drinking, sleep duration and wake after sleep onset: findings from the American time use survey. *British Journal of Nutrition*, 127(12): 1–10.

128. Chung, N., Bin, Y.S., Cistulli, P.A. & Chow, C.M. (2020). Does the proximity of meals to bedtime influence the sleep of young adults? A cross-sectional survey of university students. *International Journal of Environmental Research and Public Health*, 17(8): 2677.

129. Crispim, C.A., Zimberg, I.Z., Dos Reis, B.G., Diniz, R.M., Tufik, S. & De Mello, M.T. (2011). Relationship between food intake and sleep pattern in healthy individuals. *Journal of Clinical Sleep Medicine*, 7(6): 659–664.

130. Uçar, C., Özgöçer, T. & Yıldız, S. (2021). Effects of late-night eating of easily-or slowly-digestible meals on sleep, hypothalamo-pituitary-adrenal axis, and autonomic nervous system in healthy young males. *Stress Health*, 37(4): 640–649.

131. Chan, V. & Lo, K. (2022). Efficacy of dietary supplements on improving sleep quality: a systematic review and meta-analysis. *Postgraduate Medical Journal*, 98(1158): 285–293.

132. Poursaleh, Z., Khodadoost, M., Vahedi, E., Ahmadian-Attari, M., Jafari, M. & Poursaleh, E. (2021). A review of available herbal medicine options for the treatment of chronic insomnia. *Pakistan Journal of Medical and Health Sciences*, 15(5): 1589–1598.

133. Ell, J., Schmid, S.R., Benz, F. & Spille, L. (2023). Complementary and alternative treatments for insomnia disorder: a systematic umbrella review. *Journal of Sleep Research*, 32(6): e13979.

134. Sutanto, C.N., Loh, W.W. & Kim, J.E. (2022). The impact of tryptophan supplementation on sleep quality: a systematic review, meta-analysis, and meta-regression. *Nutrition Reviews*, 80(2): 306–316.

135. Choi, K., Lee, Y.J., Park, S., Je, N.K. & Suh, H.S. (2022). Efficacy of melatonin for chronic insomnia: systematic reviews and meta-analyses. *Sleep Medicine Reviews*, 66: 101692.

136. Händel, M.N., Andersen, H.K., Ussing, A., *et al.* (2023). The short-term and long-term adverse effects of melatonin treatment in children and adolescents: a systematic review and GRADE assessment. *EClinicalMedicine*, 61: 102083.

137. Tuft, C., Matar, E., Menczel Schrire, Z., Grunstein, R.R., Yee, B.J. & Hoyos, C.M. (2023). Current insights into the risks of using melatonin as a treatment for sleep disorders in older adults. *Clinical Interventions in Aging*, 18: 49–59.

138. Sateia, M.J., Buysse, D.J., Krystal, A.D., Neubauer, D.N. & Heald, J.L. (2017). Clinical practice guideline for the pharmacologic treatment of chronic insomnia in adults: an American Academy of Sleep Medicine Clinical Practice Guideline. *Journal of Clinical Sleep Medicine*, 13(2): 307–349.

139. Komada, Y., Okajima, I. & Kuwata, T. (2020). The effects of milk and dairy products on sleep: a systematic review. *International Journal of Environmental Research and Public Health*, 17(24): 9440.

140. Panurywanti, E., Wiboworini, B. & Indarto, D. (2021). The effect of banana dose and duration on the decrease of sleep disorders in the elderly. *Journal of Medical and Allied Sciences*, 11: 71.

141. Lin, H.H., Tsai, P.S., Fang, S.C. & Liu, J.F. (2011). Effect of kiwifruit consumption on sleep quality in adults with sleep problems. *Asia Pacific Journal of Clinical Nutrition*, 20(2): 169–174.

142. Losso, J., Finley, J., Karki, N., *et al.* (2018). Pilot study of the tart cherry juice for the treatment of insomnia and investigation of mechanisms. *American Journal of Therapeutics*, 25: e194–e201.

143. Vallat, R., Berry, S.E., Tsereteli, N., *et al.* (2022). How people wake up is associated with previous night's sleep together with physical activity and food intake. *Nature Communications*, 13(1): 7116.

144. McStay, M., Gabel, K., Cienfuegos, S., Ezpeleta, M., Lin, S. & Varady, K.A. (2021). Intermittent fasting and sleep: a review of human trials. *Nutrients*, 13(10): 3489.

6. Social Sleep

1. Canetti, E. (1942–1994). *Records (Aufzeichnungen)*. Carl Hanser Verlag.
2. Crittenden, A.N., Samson, D.R., Herlosky, K.N., Mabulla, I.A., Mabulla, A.Z.P. & McKenna, J.J. (2018). Infant co-sleeping patterns and maternal sleep quality among Hadza hunter-gatherers. *Sleep Health*, 4(6): 527–534.
3. Ibid.
4. Marlowe, F.W. (2004). Mate preferences among Hadza hunter-gatherers. *Human Nature*, 15(4): 365–376.
5. Bajoghli, H., Keshavarzi, Z., Mohammadi, M.R., *et al.* (2014). 'I love you more than I can stand!' Romantic love, symptoms of depression and anxiety, and sleep complaints are related among young adults. *International Journal of Psychiatry in Clinical Practice*, 18(3): 169–174.
6. Brand, S., Foell, S., Bajoghli, H., *et al.* (2015). 'Tell me, how bright your hypomania is, and I tell you, if you are happily in love!': among young adults in love, bright side hypomania is related to reduced depression and anxiety, and better sleep quality. *International Journal of Psychiatry in Clinical Practice*, 19(1): 24–31.
7. Kuula, L., Partonen, T. & Pesonen, A.K. (2020). Emotions relating to romantic love-further disruptors of adolescent sleep. *Sleep Health*, 6(2): 159–165.
8. Bode, A. & Kuula, L. (2021). Romantic love and sleep variations: potential proximate mechanisms and evolutionary functions. *Biology (Basel)*, 10(9): 923. doi: 10.3390/biology10090923.
9. Sundelin, T., Lekander, M., Kecklund, G., Van Someren, E.J., Olsson, A. & Axelsson, J. (2013). Cues of fatigue: effects of sleep deprivation on facial appearance. *Sleep*, 36(9): 1355–1360.
10. Doi, Y., Minowa, M. & Tango, T. (2003). Impact and correlates of poor sleep quality in Japanese white-collar employees. *Sleep*, 26(4): 467–471.

11. Guo, X., Meng, Y., Lian, H., *et al.* (2023). Marital status and living apart affect sleep quality in male military personnel: a study of the China's Navy during COVID-19. *Frontiers in Psychiatry*, 14: 1178235.

12. Barclay, N.L., Eley, T.C., Buysse, D.J., Maughan, B. & Gregory, A.M. (2012). Nonshared environmental influences on sleep quality: a study of monozygotic twin differences. *Behavior Genetics*, 42(2): 234–244.

13. Stafford, M., Bendayan, R., Tymoszuk, U. & Kuh, D. (2017). Social support from the closest person and sleep quality in later life: Evidence from a British birth cohort study. *Journal of Psychosomatic Research*, 98: 1–9.

14. Gordon, A.M. & Chen, S. (2014). The role of sleep in interpersonal conflict: do sleepless nights mean worse fights? *Social Psychological and Personality Science*, 5(2): 168–175.

15. Liu, Y., Lin, W., Liu, C., *et al.* (2016). Memory consolidation reconfigures neural pathways involved in the suppression of emotional memories. *Nature Communications*, 7: 13375.

16. Rose, S., Berg-Cross, L. & Crowell, N.A. (2017). Sleep and psychological abuse among cohabiting couples: a pilot study. *Partner Abuse*, 8(4): 347–360.

17. Field, T., Diego, M., Pelaez, M., Deeds, O. & Delgado, J. Breakup distress in university students. *Adolescence*, 44(176): 705–727.

18. Lancel, M., Stroebe, M. & Eisma, M.C. (2020). Sleep disturbances in bereavement: a systematic review. *Sleep Medicine Reviews*, 53: 101331.

19. Pankhurst, F.P. & Horne, J.A. (1994). The influence of bed partners on movement during sleep. *Sleep.* 17(4): 308–315.

20. Dittami, J., Keckeis, M., Machatschke, I., Katina, S., Zeitlhofer, J. & Kloesch, G. (2007). Sex differences in the reactions to sleeping in pairs versus sleeping alone in humans. *Sleep and Biological Rhythms*, 5(4): 271–276.

21. Spiegelhalder, K., Regen, W., Siemon, F., *et al.* (2017). Your place or mine? Does the sleep location matter in young couples? *Behavioral Sleep Medicine*, 15(2): 87–96.

22. Drews, H.J., Wallot, S., Brysch, P., *et al.* (2020). Bed-sharing in couples is associated with increased and stabilized REM sleep and sleep-stage synchronization. *Frontiers in Psychiatry*, 11: 583.

23. Gravett, N., Bhagwandin, A., Lyamin, O.I., Siegel, J.M. & Manger, P.R. (2017). Sociality affects REM sleep episode duration under controlled laboratory conditions in the Rock Hyrax, *Procavia capensis*. *Frontiers in Neuroanatomy*, 11: 105.

24. Drews, H.J., Wallot, S., Brysch, P., *et al.* (2020). Bed-sharing in couples is associated with increased and stabilized REM sleep and sleep-stage synchronization. *Frontiers in Psychiatry*, 11: 583.

25. Ibid.

26. Pérez, A., Carreiras, M. & Duñabeitia, J.A. (2017). Brain-to-brain entrainment: EEG interbrain synchronization while speaking and listening. *Scientific Reports*, 7(1): 4190.

27. Volkovich, E., Ben-Zion, H., Karny, D., Meiri, G. & Tikotzky, L. (2015). Sleep patterns of co-sleeping and solitary sleeping infants and mothers: a longitudinal study. *Sleep Medicine*, 16(11): 1305–1312.

28. Krahn, L.E., Tovar, M.D. & Miller, B. (2015). Are pets in the bedroom a problem? *Mayo Clinic Proceedings*, 90(12): 1663–1665.

29. Patel, S.I., Miller, B.W., Kosiorek, H.E., Parish, J.M., Lyng, P.J. & Krahn, L.E. (2017). The effect of dogs on human sleep in the home sleep environment. *Mayo Clinic Proceedings*, 92(9): 1368–1372.

30. Hoedlmoser, K., Kloesch, G., Wiater, A. & Schabus, M. (2010). Self-reported sleep patterns, sleep problems, and behavioral problems among school children aged 8-11 years. *Somnologie (Berlin)*, 14(1): 23–31.

31. Kalmbach, D.A., Arnedt, J.T., Pillai, V. & Ciesla, J.A. (2015). The impact of sleep on female sexual response and behavior: a pilot study. *Journal of Sexual Medicine*, 12(5): 1221–1232.

32. Kohn, T.P., Kohn, J.R., Haney, N.M., Pastuszak, A.W. & Lipshultz, L.I. (2020). The effect of sleep on men's health. *Translational Andrology and Urolology*, 9(Suppl 2): S178–S185.

33. Rodriguez, K.M., Kohn, T.P., Kohn, J.R., *et al.* (2020). Shift work sleep disorder and night shift work significantly impair erectile function. *Journal of Sexual Medicine*, 17(9): 1687–1693.

34. Pastuszak, A.W., Moon, Y.M., Scovell, J., *et al.* (2017). Poor sleep quality predicts hypogonadal symptoms and sexual dysfunction in male nonstandard shift workers. *Urology*, 102: 121–125.

35. Pakzad, R., Safiri, S. Re: Pastuszak *et al.*: Poor sleep quality predicts hypogonadal symptoms and sexual dysfunction in male – nonstandard shift workers: methodological issues to avoid prediction fallacy. *Urology*, 102: 121–125.

36. Lastella, M., O'Mullan, C., Paterson, J.L. & Reynolds, A.C. (2019). Sex and sleep: perceptions of sex as a sleep promoting behavior in the general adult population. *Frontiers in Public Health*, 7: 33.

37. Blair, K.L., Cappell, J. & Pukall, C.F. (2018). Not all orgasms were created equal: differences in frequency and satisfaction of orgasm experiences by sexual activity in same-sex versus mixed-sex relationships. *Journal of Sex Research*, 55: 719–733.

38. Sprajcer, M., O'Mullan, C., Reynolds, A., Paterson, J.L., Bachmann, A. & Lastella, M. (2022). Sleeping together: understanding the association between relationship type, sexual activity, and sleep. *Sleep Science*, 15(Spec 1): 80–88.

39. Nuno, S.M. (2017). Let's talk about sex: the importance of open communication about sexuality before and during relationships. In N.R. Silton (ed.) *Family Dynamics and Romantic Relationships in a Changing Society*. IGI Global, pp. 47–61.

40. Brody, S. & Krüger, T.H. (2006). The post-orgasmic prolactin increase following intercourse is greater than following masturbation and suggests greater satiety. *Biological Psychology*, 71: 312–315.

41. Lipschitz, D.L., Kuhn, R., Kinney, A.Y., Grewen, K., Donaldson, G.W. & Nakamura, Y. (2015). An exploratory study of the effects of mind–body interventions targeting sleep on salivary oxytocin levels in cancer survivors. *Integrative Cancer Therapies*, 14:366–380.

42. Kim, D.A., Benjamin, E.J., Fowler, J.H. & Christakis, N.A. (2016). Social connectedness is associated with fibrinogen level in a human social network. *Proceedings of the Royal Society B: Biological Sciences*, 283: 20160958.

43. Fedurek, P., Lehmann, J., Lacroix, L., *et al.* (2023). Status does not predict stress among Hadza hunter-gatherer men. *Scientific Reports*, 13(1): 1327.

44. Stalder, T. *et al.* (2017). Stress-related and basic determinants of hair cortisol in humans: a meta-analysis. *Psychoneuroendocrinology*, 77: 261–274.

45. Tavernier, R. & Willoughby, T. (2015). A longitudinal examination of the bidirectional association between sleep problems and social ties at university: the mediating role of emotion regulation. *Journal of Youth and Adolescence*, 44(2): 317–330.

46. Ben Simon, E. & Walker, M.P. (2018). Sleep loss causes social withdrawal and loneliness. *Nature Communications*, 9(1): 3146.

47. Kurina, L.M., Knutson, K.L., Hawkley, L.C., Cacioppo, J.T., Lauderdale, D.S. & Ober, C. (2011). Loneliness is associated with sleep fragmentation in a communal society. *Sleep*, 34(11): 1519–1526.

48. Aanes, M.M., Hetland, J., Pallesen, S. & Mittelmark, M.B. (2011). Does loneliness mediate the stress-sleep quality relation? The Hordaland Health Study. *International Psychogeriatrics*, 23(6): 994–1002.

49. Cheng, G.H., Malhotra, R., Chan, A., Østbye, & Lo, J.C. (2018). Weak social networks and restless sleep interrelate through depressed mood among elderly. *Quality of Life Research*, 27(10): 2517–2524.

50. Kent de Grey, R.G., Uchino, B.N., Trettevik, R., Cronan, S. & Hogan, J.N. (2018). Social support and sleep: a meta-analysis. *Health Psychology*, 37(8): 787–798.

51. Mesas, A.E., Peppard, P.E., Hale, L., Friedman, E.M., Nieto, F.J. & Hagen, E.W. Individuals' perceptions of social support from family and friends are associated with lower risk of sleep complaints and short sleep duration. *Sleep Health*, 6(1): 110–116.

52. Janssens, L., Giemsch, L., Schmitz, R., Street, M., Van Dongen, S. & Crombé, P. (2018). A new look at an old dog: Bonn-Oberkassel reconsidered. *Journal of Archaeological Science*, 92: 126–138.

53. Lahtinen, M., Clinnick, D., Mannermaa, K., Salonen, J.S. & Viranta, S. (2021). Excess protein enabled dog domestication during severe Ice Age winters. *Scientific Reports*, 11(1): 7.

54. Mein, G. & Grant, R. (2018). A cross-sectional exploratory analysis between pet ownership, sleep, exercise, health and neighbourhood perceptions: the Whitehall II cohort study. *BMC Geriatrics*, 18(1): 176.

55. Mičková, E., Machová, K., Daďová, K. & Svobodová, I. (2019). Does dog ownership affect physical activity, sleep, and self-reported health in older adults? *International Journal of Environmental Research and Public Health*, 16(18): 3355.

56. Van Egmond, L.T., Titova, O.E., Lindberg, E., Fall, T. & Benedict, C. (2021). Association between pet ownership and sleep in the Swedish Cardio Pulmonary bioImage Study (SCAPIS). *Scientific Reports*, 11(1): 7468.

57. Medlin, K. & Wisnieski, L. (2023). The association of pet ownership and sleep quality and sleep disorders in United States. *Human-Animal Interactions*, March.

58. Fedurek, P., Lehmann, J., Lacroix, L., *et al.* (2023). Status does not predict stress among Hadza hunter-gatherer men. *Scientific Reports*, 13(1): 1327.

59. Rigó, M., Dragano, N., Wahrendorf, M., Siegrist, J. & Lunau, T. (2021). Work stress on rise? Comparative analysis of trends in work stressors using the European working conditions survey. *International Archives of Occupational and Environmental Health*, 94(3): 459–474.

60. Van Laethem, M., Beckers, D.C.J., Kompier, M.A.J., *et al.* (2015). Bidirectional relations between work-related stress, sleep quality and perseverative cognition. *Journal of Psychosomatic Research*, 79(5): 391–398.

61. Calem, M., Bisla, J., Begum, A., *et al.* (2012). Increased prevalence of insomnia and changes in hypnotics use in England over 15 years: analysis of the 1993, 2000, and 2007 National Psychiatric Morbidity Surveys. *Sleep*, 35(3): 377–384.

62. Linton, S.J. (2004). Does work stress predict insomnia? A prospective study. *British Journal of Health Psychology*, 9(Pt 2): 127–136.

63. Reynolds, A.C., Coenen, P., Lechat, B., *et al.* (2023). Insomnia and workplace productivity loss among young working adults: a prospective observational study of clinical sleep disorders in a community cohort. *Medical Journal of Australia*, 219(3): 107–112.

64. Shahly, V., Berglund, P.A., Coulouvrat, C. *et al.* (2012). The associations of insomnia with costly workplace accidents and errors: results from the America Insomnia Survey. *Archives of General Psychiatry*, 69(10): 1054–1063.

65. Vega-Escaño, J., Porcel-Gálvez, A.M., Diego-Cordero, R., Romero-Sánchez, J.M., Romero-Saldaña, M. & Barrientos-Trigo, S. (2020). Insomnia interventions in the workplace: a systematic review and meta-analysis. *International Journal of Environmental Research and Public Health*, 17(17): 6401.

66. Scott, B.A. & Judge, T.A. (2006). Insomnia, emotions, and job satisfaction: a multilevel study. *Journal of Management*, 32(5): 622–645.

7. Stimulating Sleep

1. Trollope, A. (1855). *The Warden*. Longman.

2. Fredholm, B.B. (2011). Notes on the history of caffeine use. *Handbook of Experimental Pharmacology*, (200): 1–9.

3. O'Callaghan, F., Muurlink, O. & Reid, N. (2018). Effects of caffeine on sleep quality and daytime functioning. *Risk Management and Healthcare Policy*, 11: 263–271.

4. Drake, C., Roehrs, T., Shambroom, J. & Roth, T. (2013). Caffeine effects on sleep taken 0, 3, or 6 hours before going to bed. *Journal of Clinical Sleep Medicine*, 9(11): 1195–1200.

5. Karacan, I., Thornby, J.I., Anch, M., Booth, G.H., Williams, R.L. & Salis, P.J. (1976). Dose-related sleep disturbances induced by coffee and caffeine. *Clinical Pharmacology and Therapeutics*, 20(6): 682–689.

6. Janson, C., Gislason, T., De Backer, W., *et al.* (1995). Prevalence of sleep disturbances among young adults in three European countries. *Sleep*, 18(7): 589–597.

7. Sanchez-Ortuno, M., Moore, N., Taillard, J., *et al.* (2005). Sleep duration and caffeine consumption in a French middle-aged working population. *Sleep Medicine*, 6(3): 247–251.

8. Weibel, J., Lin, Y.S., Landolt, H.P., *et al.* (2021). The impact of daily caffeine intake on nighttime sleep in young adult men. *Scientific Reports*, 11(1): 4668.

9. Bonnet, M.H. & Arand, D.L. (1992). Caffeine use as a model of acute and chronic insomnia. *Sleep*, 15(6): 526–536.

10. O'Callaghan, F., Muurlink, O. & Reid, N. (2018). Effects of caffeine on sleep quality and daytime functioning. *Risk Management and Healthcare Policy*, 11: 263–271.

11. Bodenmann, S., Hohoff, C., Freitag, C., *et al.* (2012). Polymorphisms of ADORA2A modulate psychomotor vigilance and the effects of caffeine on neurobehavioural performance and sleep EEG after sleep deprivation. *British Journal of Pharmacology*, 165(6): 1904–1913.

12. Clark, I. & Landolt, H.P. (2017). Coffee, caffeine, and sleep: a systematic review of epidemiological studies and randomized controlled trials. *Sleep Medicine Reviews*, 31: 70–78.

13. Tushingham, S., Ardura, D., Eerkens, J.W., Palazoglu, M., Shahbaz, S. & Oliver, O. (2013). Hunter-gatherer tobacco smoking: earliest evidence from the Pacific Northwest Coast of North America. *Journal of Archaeological Science*, 40 (2): 1397–1407.

14. Philips, J.E. (1983). African smoking and pipes. *Journal of African History*, 24(3): 303–319.

15. Laufer, B., Hambley, W.D. & Linton, R. (1930). *Tobacco and its use in Africa*. Field Museum of Natural History.

16. Garcia, A.N. & Salloum, I.M. (2015). Polysomnographic sleep disturbances in nicotine, caffeine, alcohol, cocaine, opioid, and cannabis use: a focused review. *American Journal of Addictions*, 24(7): 590–598.

17. AlRyalat, S.A., Kussad, S., El Khatib, O., *et al.* (2021). Assessing the effect of nicotine dose in cigarette smoking on sleep quality. *Sleep and Breathing*, 25(3): 1319–1324.

18. Benowitz, N.L. (1997). The role of nicotine in smoking-related cardiovascular disease. *Preventive Medicine*, 26(4): 412–417.

19. Caviness, C.M., Anderson, B.J. & Stein, M.D. (2019). Impact of nicotine and other stimulants on sleep in young adults. *Journal of Addiction Medicine*, 13(3): 209–214.

20. Jaehne, A., Loessl, B., Bárkai, Z., Riemann, D. & Hornyak, M. (2009). Effects of nicotine on sleep during consumption, withdrawal and replacement therapy. *Sleep Medicine Reviews*, 13(5): 363–377.

21. Dugas, E.N., Sylvestre, M.P., O'Loughlin, E.K., *et al.* (2017). Nicotine dependence and sleep quality in young adults. *Addictive Behaviors*, 65: 154–160.

22. Branstetter, S.A., Horton, W.J., Mercincavage, M. & Buxton, O.M. (2016). Severity of nicotine addiction and disruptions in sleep mediated by early awakenings. *Nicotine & Tobacco Research*, 18(12): 2252–2259.

23. Teofilo, L. (2008). *Medications and their Effects on Sleep. Sleep Medicine: Essentials and Review*. Oxford University Press, pp. 35–72.

24. Knight, J.K., Salali, G.D., Sikka, G., Derkx, I., Keestra, S.M. & Chaudhary, N. (2021). Quantifying patterns of alcohol consumption and its effects on health and wellbeing among BaYaka hunter-gatherers: a mixed-methods cross-sectional study. *PLoS One*, 16(10): e0258384.

25. Stahre, M., Naimi, T., Brewer, R. & Holt, J. (2006). Measuring average alcohol consumption: the impact of including binge drinks in quantity-frequency calculations. *Addiction*, 101(12): 1711–1718.

26. Landolt, H.P. & Gillin, J.C. (2001). Sleep abnormalities during abstinence in alcohol-dependent patients. Aetiology and management. *CNS Drugs*, 15(5): 413–425.

27. Devenney, L.E., Coyle, K.B., Roth, T. & Verster J.C. (2019). Sleep after heavy alcohol consumption and physical activity levels during alcohol hangover. *Journal of Clinical Medicine*, 8(5): 752.

28. Brower, K.J., Aldrich, M.S., Robinson, E.A., Zucker, R.A. & Greden, J.F. (2001). Insomnia, self-medication, and relapse to alcoholism. *American Journal of Psychiatry*, 158(3): 399–404.

29. Helaakoski, V., Kaprio, J., Hublin, C., Ollila, H.M. & Latvala, A. (2022). Alcohol use and poor sleep quality: a longitudinal twin study across 36 years. *SLEEP Advances*, 3(1): 1–10.

30. Landolt, H.P. & Gillin, J.C. (2001). Sleep abnormalities during abstinence in alcohol-dependent patients. Aetiology and management. *CNS Drugs*, 15(5): 413–425.

31. Russo, E.B., Jiang, H.E., Li, X., *et al.* (2008). Phytochemical and genetic analyses of ancient cannabis from Central Asia. *Journal of Experimental* Botany, 59(15): 4171–4182.

32. Roulette, C. & Hewlett, B. (2018). Patterns of cannabis use among Congo Basin hunter-gatherers. *Journal of Ethnobiology*. 38(4): 517–532.

33. Volkow, N.D., Baler, R.D., Compton, W.M. & Weiss, S.R. (2014). Adverse health effects of marijuana use. *New England Journal of Medicine*, 370(23): 2219–2227.

34. Budney, A.J. & Hughes, J.R. (2006). The cannabis withdrawal syndrome. *Current Opinion in Psychiatry*, 19(3): 233–238.

35. Velzeboer, R., Malas, A., Boerkoel P., *et al.* (2022). Cannabis dosing and administration for sleep: a systematic review. *Sleep*, 15: zsac218.

36. Brunt, T.M., Van Genugten, M., Höner-Snoeken, K., Van de Velde, M.J. & Niesink, R.J. (2014). Therapeutic satisfaction and subjective effects of different strains of pharmaceutical-grade cannabis. *Journal of Clinical Psychopharmacology*, 34(3): 344–349.

37. Schierenbeck, T., Riemann, D., Berger, M. & Hornyak, M. (2008). Effect of illicit recreational drugs upon sleep: cocaine, ecstasy and marijuana. *Sleep Medicine Reviews*, 12(5): 381–389.

38. Volkow, N.D., Baler, R.D., Compton, W.M. & Weiss, S.R. (2014). Adverse health effects of marijuana use. *New England Journal of Medicine*, 370(23): 2219–2227.

39. Gertsch, J. (2018). The Intricate Influence of the placebo effect on medical cannabis and cannabinoids. *Medical Cannabis and Cannabinoids*, 1(1): 60–64.

40. Williamson, S., Gossop, M., Powis, B., Griffiths, P., Fountain, J. & Strang, J. (1997). Adverse effects of stimulant drugs in a community sample of drug users. *Drug and Alcohol Dependence*, 44(2-3): 87–94.

41. Irwin, M.R., Bjurstrom, M.F. & Olmstead, R. (2016). Polysomnographic measures of sleep in cocaine dependence and alcohol dependence: implications for age-related loss of slow wave, stage 3 sleep. *Addiction*, 111(6): 1084–1092.

42. Liu, Y., Williamson, V., Setlow, B., Cottler, L.B. & Knackstedt, L.A. (2018). The importance of considering polysubstance use: lessons from cocaine research. *Drug and Alcohol Dependence*, 192: 16–28.

43. Wheeler, P.B., Dogan, J.N., Stevens-Watkins, D. & Stoops, W.W. (2021). Sleep time differs among people who co-use cocaine and cannabis compared to people who only use cocaine. *Pharmacology Biochemistry and Behavior*, 201: 173109.

44. Williamson, S., Gossop, M., Powis, B., Griffiths, P., Fountain, J. & Strang, J. (1997). Adverse effects of stimulant drugs in a community sample of drug users. *Drug and Alcohol Dependence*, 44(2-3): 87–94.

45. Khazaie, H., Jalali, A., Jozani, Y., Moradi, S., Heydarpou,r F. & Khaledi-Paveh, B. (2016). Comparative study on sleep quality and disorders in opiate and methamphetamine users. *Heroin Addiction and Related Clinical Problems*, 18(6): 21–28.

46. Rechtschaffen, A. & Maron, L. (1964). The effect of amphetamine on the sleep cycle. *Electroencephalography and Clinical Neurophysiology*, 16: 438–445.

47. Verheyden, S.L., Henry, J.A. & Curran, H.V. (2003). Acute, subacute and long-term subjective consequences of 'ecstasy' (MDMA) consumption in 430 regular users. *Human Psychopharmacology*, 18(7): 507–517.

48. Gouzoulis, E., Steiger, A., Ensslin, M., Kovar, A. & Hermle, L. (1992). Sleep EEG effects of 3,4-methylenedioxyethamphetamine (MDE; 'eve') in healthy volunteers. *Biological Psychiatry*, 32(12): 1108–1117.

49. Ponte, L., Jerome, L., Hamilton, S., *et al.* (2021). Sleep quality improvements after MDMA-assisted psychotherapy for the treatment of posttraumatic stress disorder. *Journal of Traumatic Stress*, 34(4): 851–863.

50. Watson, R., Hartmann, E. & Schildkraut, J.J. (1972). Amphetamine withdrawal: affective state, sleep patterns, and MHPG excretion. *American Journal of Psychiatry*, 129(3): 263–269.

51. Ardani, A.R., Saghebi, S.A., Nahidi, M. & Zeynalian, F. (2016). Does abstinence resolve poor sleep quality in former methamphetamine dependents? *Sleep Science*, 9(3): 255–260.

8. Relax!

1. Reverdy, P. (1945). *Plupart du temps. Poèmes 1915-1922*. Gallimard.

2. Wiessner, P.W. (2014). Embers of society: firelight talk among the Ju/'hoansi Bushmen. *Proceedings of the National Academy of Sciences USA*, 111(39): 14027–14035.

3. Su, H., Xiao, L., Ren, Y., Xie, H. & Sun, X.H. (2021). Effects of mindful breathing combined with sleep-inducing exercises in patients with insomnia. *World Journal of Clinical Cases*, 9(29): 8740–8748.

4. Holmes, E.A. & Mathews, A. (2010). Mental imagery in emotion and emotional disorders. *Clinical Psychology Review*, 30: 349–362.

5. Nguyen, J. & Brymer, E. (2018). Nature-based guided imagery as an intervention for state anxiety. *Frontiers in Psychology*, 9: 1858.

6. Lawton, E., Brymer, E., Clough, P. & Denovan, A. (2017). The relationship between the physical activity environment, nature relatedness, anxiety, and the psychological well-being benefits of regular exercisers. *Frontiers in Psychology*, 8: 1058.

7. Nguyen, J. & Brymer, E. (2018). Nature-based guided imagery as an intervention for state anxiety. *Frontiers in Psychology*, 9: 1858.

8. Gong, H., Ni, C.X., Liu, Y.Z., *et al.* (2016). Mindfulness meditation for insomnia: a meta-analysis of randomized controlled trials. *Journal of Psychosomatic Research*, 89: 1–6.

9. Wang, Y., Wang, F., Zheng, W., *et al.* (2020). Mindfulness-based interventions for insomnia: a meta-analysis of randomized controlled trials. *Behavioral Sleep Medicine*, 18(1): 1–9.

9. Working with Hours

1. Nietzsche, F.W. (1883–1892). *Thus Spoke Zarathustra: A Book for All and None*. Ernst Schmeitzner.

2. Buysse, D.J., Reynolds, C.F. 3rd, Monk, T.H., Berman, S.R. & Kupfer, D.J. (1989). The Pittsburgh Sleep Quality Index: a new instrument for psychiatric practice and research. *Psychiatry Research*, 28(2): 193–213.

3. Brindle, R.C., Yu, L., Buysse, D.J. & Hall, M.H. (2019). Empirical derivation of cutoff values for the sleep health metric and its relationship to cardiometabolic morbidity: results from the midlife in the United States (MIDUS) study. *Sleep*, 42(9): zsz116.

4. Hirshkowitz, M., Whiton, K., Albert, S.M., *et al.* (2015). National Sleep Foundation's updated sleep duration recommendations: final report. *Sleep Health*, 1(4): 233–243.

5. Van Den Berg, J.F., Van Rooij. F.J., Vos, H., *et al.* (2008). Disagreement between subjective and actigraphic measures of sleep duration in a population-based study of elderly persons. *Journal of Sleep Research*, 17(3): 295–302.

6. Lehrer, H.M., Yao, Z., Krafty, R.T., *et al.* (2022). Comparing polysomnography, actigraphy, and sleep diary in the home environment: the Study of Women's Health Across the Nation (SWAN) Sleep Study. *Sleep Advances*, 3(1): zpac001.

7. Hesse, H. (1943). *Das Glasperlenspiel*. Fretz & Wasmuth.

8. Du Laurens, M.A. (1599). *A discourse of the preservation of the sight; of melancholike diseases; of rheumes, and of old age*, translated by R. Surphlet. Felix Kingston for Ralph Iacson, London.

9. Poyares, D., Guilleminault, C., Ohayon, M. & Tufik, S. (2004). Chronic benzodiazepine usage and withdrawal in insomnia patients. *Journal of Psychiatric Research*, 38: 327–334.

10. Crowe, S.F. & Stranks, E.K. (2018). The residual medium and long-term cognitive effects of benzodiazepine use: an updated meta-analysis. *Archives of Clinical Neuropsychology*, 33(7): 901–911.

11. Puustinen, J., Lähteenmäki, R., Polo-Kantola, P., *et al.* (2014). Effect of withdrawal from long-term use of temazepam, zopiclone or zolpidem as hypnotic agents on cognition in older adults. *European Journal of Clinical Pharmacology*, 70(3): 319–329.

12. Moore, T.J. & Mattison, D.R. (2017). Adult utilization of psychiatric drugs and differences by sex, age, and race. *JAMA Internal Medicine*, 177(2): 274–275.

13. Bachhuber, M.A., Hennessy, S., Cunningham, C.O. & Starrels, J.L. (2016). Increasing benzodiazepine prescriptions and overdose mortality in the United States, 1996–2013. *American Journal of Public Health*, 106(4): 686–688.

14. Soyka, M., Wild, I., Caulet, B., Leontiou, C., Lugoboni, F. & Hajak, G. (2023. Long-term use of benzodiazepines in chronic insomnia: a European perspective. *Frontiers in Psychiatry*, 14: 1212028.

15. Davies, J., Rae, T.C. & Montagu, L. (2017). Long-term benzodiazepine and Z-drugs use in England: a survey of general practice [corrected]. *British Journal of General Practice*, 67(662): e609–e613.

16. Van Straten, A., Van der Zweerde, T., Kleiboer, A., Cuijpers, P., Morin, C. & Lancee, J. (2018). Cognitive and behavioral therapies in the treatment of insomnia: a meta-analysis. *Sleep Medicine Reviews*, 38: 3–16.

17. Morin, C.M., Hauri, P.J., Espie, C.A., Spielman, A.J., Buysse, D.J. & Bootzin, R.R. (1999). Nonpharmacologic treatment of chronic insomnia. An American Academy of Sleep Medicine review. *Sleep*, 22(8): 1134–1156.

18. Van de Laar, M., Pevernagie, D., Van Mierlo, P. & Overeem, S. (2015). Psychiatric comorbidity and aspects of cognitive coping negatively predict outcome in cognitive behavioral treatment of psychophysiological insomnia. *Behavioral Sleep Medicine*, 13: 140–156.

19. Ibid.

20. Ibid.

21. McCurry, S.M., Guthrie, K.A., Morin, C.M., *et al.* (2016). Telephone-based cognitive behavioral therapy for insomnia in perimenopausal and postmenopausal women with vasomotor symptoms: a MsFLASH randomized clinical trial. *JAMA Internal Medicine*, 176(7): 913–920.

22. Drake, C.L., Kalmbach, D.A., Arnedt, J.T., *et al.* (2019). Treating chronic insomnia in postmenopausal women: a randomized

clinical trial comparing cognitive-behavioral therapy for insomnia, sleep restriction therapy, and sleep hygiene education. *Sleep*, 42(2): zsy217.

23. Maurer, L.F., Schneider, J., Miller, C.B., Espie, C.A. & Kyle, S.D. The clinical effects of sleep restriction therapy for insomnia: a meta-analysis of randomised controlled trials. *Sleep Medicine Reviews*, 58: 101493.

24. Ibid.

25. Maurer, L.F., Espie, C.A., Omlin, X., Emsley, R. & Kyle, S.D. The effect of sleep restriction therapy for insomnia on sleep pressure and arousal: a randomized controlled mechanistic trial. *Sleep*, 45(1): zsab223.

26. Cain, N., Richardson, C., Bartel, K., Whittall, H., Reeks, J. & Gradisar, M. (2022). A randomised controlled dismantling trial of sleep restriction therapies for chronic insomnia disorder in middle childhood: effects on sleep and anxiety, and possible contraindications. *Journal of Sleep Research*, 17: e13658.

27. Miller, C.B., Espie, C.A., Epstein, D.R., *et al.* (2014). The evidence base of sleep restriction therapy for treating insomnia disorder. *Sleep Medicine Reviews*, 18(5): 415–424.

28. Verreault, M.D., Granger, É., Neveu, X., Delage, J.P., Bastien, C.H. & Vallières, A. (2023). The effectiveness of stimulus control in cognitive behavioural therapy for insomnia in adults: A systematic review and network meta-analysis. *Journal of Sleep Research*, 16: e14008.

29. Bootzin, R.R. (1972). Stimulus control treatment for insomnia. *Proceedings of the American Psychological Association*, 7: 395–396.

30. Verreault, M.D., Granger, É., Neveu, X., Delage, J.P., Bastien, C.H. & Vallières, A. (2023). The effectiveness of stimulus control in cognitive behavioural therapy for insomnia in adults: A systematic review and network meta-analysis. *Journal of Sleep Research*, 16: e14008.

10. Clashing Clocks and Nightly Ghosts

1. Euginedes, J. (2011). *The Marriage Plot*. Farrar, Straus and Giroux.
2. Hawthorne, N. (1850). *The Scarlet Letter: A Romance*. Boston. Tickner, Reed and Fields.
3. American Academy of Sleep Medicine. (2014). *The International Classification of Sleep Disorders – Third Edition* (*ICSD-3*). American Academy of Sleep Medicine.
4. Valli, K. & Revonsuo, A. (2009). The threat simulation theory in light of recent empirical evidence: a review. *American Journal of Psychology*, 122: 17–38.
5. Danielsson, K., Markström, A., Broman, J.E., Von Knorring, L. & Jansson-Fröjmark, M. (2016). Delayed sleep phase disorder in a Swedish cohort of adolescents and young adults: prevalence and associated factors. *Chronobiology International*, 33(10): 1331–1339.
6. Micic, G., de Bruyn, A., Lovato, N., *et al.* (2013). The endogenous circadian temperature period length (tau) in delayed sleep phase disorder compared to good sleepers. *Journal of Sleep Research*, 22: 617–624.
7. Aoki, H., Ozeki, Y. & Yamada, N. (2001). Hypersensitivity of melatonin suppression in response to light in patients with delayed sleep phase syndrome. *Chronobiology International*, 18: 263–271.
8. Jones, C., Huang, A., Ptacek, L. & Fu, Y. (2013). Genetic basis of human circadian rhythm disorders. *Experimental Neurology*, 243: 28–33.
9. Wyatt, J. (2004). Delayed sleep phase syndrome: pathophysiology and treatment options. *Sleep*, 27: 1195–1203.
10. Ambesh, P., Shetty, V., Ambesh, S., Gupta, S.S., Kamholz, S. & Wolf, L. (2018). Jet lag: heuristics and therapeutics. *Journal of Family Medicine and Primary Care*, 7(3): 507–510.
11. Eastman C.I., Burgess H.J. (2009). How to travel the world without jet lag. *Sleep Medicine Clinics*, 4: 241–255.

12. Beaumont, M., Batéjat, D., Piérard, C., et al. (1985). Caffeine or melatonin effects on sleep and sleepiness after rapid eastward transmeridian travel. *Journal of Applied Physiology*, 96: 50–58.

13. Yellowless, D. (1878). Homicide by a somnambulist. *Journal of Mental Science*, 24: 451–458.

14. Irfan, M., Schenck, C.H. & Howell, M.J. (2017). Non-rapid eye movement sleep and overlap parasomnias. *Continuum*, 23: 1035–1050.

15. Bjorvatn, B., Grønli, J. & Pallesen, S. (2010). Prevalence of different parasomnias in the general population. *Sleep Medicine*, 11: 1031–1034.

16. Hishikawa, Y. & Shimizu, T. (1995). Physiology of REM sleep, cataplexy, and sleep paralysis. *Advance Neurology*, 67: 245–271.

17. Plazzi, G. & Montagna, P. (2002). Remitting REM sleep behavior disorder as the initial sign of multiple sclerosis. *Sleep Medicine*, 3(5): 437–439.

18. Diaconu, Ş., Falup-Pecurariu, O., Ţînţ, D. & Falup-Pecurariu, C. (2021). REM sleep behaviour disorder in Parkinson's disease (Review). *Experimental and Therapeutic Medicine*, 22(2): 812.

19. Drakatos, P. et al. (2019). NREM parasomnias: a treatment approach based upon a retrospective case series of 512 patients. *Sleep Medicine*, 53: 181–188.

20. Pressman, M. (2007). Factors that predispose, prime and precipitate NREM parasomnias in adults: clinical and forensic implications. *Sleep Medicine Reviews*, 1: 5-30.

21. Malhotra, R.K. & Avidan, A.Y. (2012). Parasomnias and their mimics. *Neurologic Clinics*, 30: 1067–1094.

22. Hurwitz, T., Mahowald, M., Schenck, C., Schluter, J. & Bundlie, S. (1991). A retrospective outcome study and review of hypnosis as treatment of adults with sleepwalking and sleep terror. *The Journal of Nervous and Mental Disease*, 179: 228–233.

23. Thompson, D.F. & Pierce, D.R. (1999). Drug-induced nightmares. *Annals of Pharmacotherapy*, 33(1): 93–98.

24. Tribl, G.G., Wetter, T.C. & Schredl, M. (2013). Dreaming under antidepressants: a systematic review on evidence in depressive patients and healthy volunteers. *Sleep Medicine Reviews*, 17(2): 133–142.

25. Brezner, I. (2011). A proposed mechanism for drug-induced nightmares. *The Science Journal of the Lander College of Arts and Sciences*, 4(2).

26. Casement, M. & Swanson, L. (2012). A meta-analysis of imagery rehearsal for post-trauma nightmares: effects on nightmare frequency, sleep quality, and post-traumatic stress. *Clinical Psychology Review*, 32: 566–574.

27. Kunze, A., Arntz, A., Morina, N., Kindt, M. & Lancee, J. (2017). Efficacy of imagery rescripting and imaginal exposure for nightmares: a randomized wait-list controlled trial. *Behaviour Research and Therapy*, 97: 14–25.

28. de Macêdo, T., Ferreira, G., de Almondes, K., Kirov, R. & Mota-Rolim, S. (2019). My dream, my rules: can lucid dreaming treat nightmares? *Frontiers in Psychology*, 10: 2618.

11. The Future of Sleep

1. Wiliams, P. (2004). *How to Be Like Walt: Capturing the Magic Every Day of Your Life*. Dearfield Beach: Health Communication.

2. Lee, J. & Finkelstein, J. (2015). Consumer sleep tracking devices: a critical review. *Studies in Health Technology and Informatics*, 210: 458–460.

3. Patel, P., Kim, J.Y. & Brooks, L.J. (2017). Accuracy of a smartphone application in estimating sleep in children. *Sleep and Breathing*, 21(2): 505–511.

4. Glazer Baron, K. et al. (2022). How are consumer sleep technology data being used to deliver behavioral sleep medicine interventions? A systematic review. *Behavioral Sleep Medicine*, 20(2): 173–187.

5. Ciman, M. & Wac, K. (2019). Smartphones as sleep duration sensors: validation of the iSenseSleep algorithm. *JMIR mHealth and uHealth.* 7(5): e11930.

6. Chiang, A.A. & Khosla, S. (2023). Consumer wearable sleep trackers: are they ready for clinical use? *Sleep Medicine Clinics*, 18(3): 311–330.

7. Fino, E. & Mazzetti, M. (2019). Monitoring healthy and disturbed sleep through smartphone applications: a review of experimental evidence. *Sleep and Breathing*, 23(1): 13–24.

8. Chinoy, E.D., Cuellar, J.A., Jameson, J.T. & Markwald, R.R. (2022). Performance of four commercial wearable sleep-tracking devices tested under unrestricted conditions at home in healthy young adults. *Nature and Science of Sleep*, 14: 493–516.

9. Baron, K.G., Abbott, S., Jao, N., Manalo, N. & Mullen, R. (2017). Orthosomnia: are some patients taking the quantified self too far? *Journal of Clinical Sleep Medicine*, 13(2): 351–354.

10. Luik, A.I., Farias Machado, P. & Espie, C.A. (2018). Delivering digital cognitive behavioral therapy for insomnia at scale: does using a wearable device to estimate sleep influence therapy? *npj Digital Medicine*, 1: 3.

11. Lee, Y.C., Lu, C.T., Cheng, W.N. & Li, H.Y. (2022). The impact of mouth-taping in mouth-breathers with mild obstructive sleep apnea: a preliminary study. *Healthcare* (Basel). 10(9): 1755.

12. Støre, S.J., Tillfors, M., Wästlund, E., Angelhoff, C., Andersson, G. & Norell-Clarke, A. (2021). The effects of a sleep robot intervention on sleep, depression and anxiety in adults with insomnia: study protocol of a randomized waitlist-controlled trial. *Contemporary Clinical Trials*, 110: 106588.

13. Riedy, S.M., Smith, M.G., Rocha, S. & Basner, M. (2021). Noise as a sleep aid: a systematic review. *Sleep Medicine Reviews*, 55: 101385.

14. Vesterager, V. (1994). Combined psychological and prosthetic management of tinnitus: a cross-sectional study of patients with severe tinnitus. *British Journal of Audiology*, 28(1): 1–11.

15. Terzano, M.G., Parrino, L., Fioriti, G., Orofiamma, B. & Depoortere, H. (1990). Modifications of sleep structure induced by increasing levels of acoustic perturbation in normal subjects. *Electroencephalography and Clinical Neurophysiology*, 76(1): 29–38.

16. Duggan, N.M., Hasdianda, M.A., Baker, O. et al. (2022). The effect of noise-masking earbuds (SleepBuds) on reported sleep quality and tension in health care shift workers: prospective single-subject design study. *JMIR Formative Research*, 6(3): e28353.

12. Balance is Key

1. Bachelard, G. (1965). *La poetique de la reverie*. Paris: Press Universitaires de France.

Index